Spontaneous abortion

Saad M. Al-araji
Nawras J. Al-Salihi

Spontaneous abortion

Main causes associated with single and recurrent abortion in Iraq

LAP LAMBERT Academic Publishing

Impressum/Imprint (nur für Deutschland/only for Germany)
Bibliografische Information der Deutschen Nationalbibliothek: Die Deutsche Nationalbibliothek verzeichnet diese Publikation in der Deutschen Nationalbibliografie; detaillierte bibliografische Daten sind im Internet über http://dnb.d-nb.de abrufbar.
Alle in diesem Buch genannten Marken und Produktnamen unterliegen warenzeichen-, marken- oder patentrechtlichem Schutz bzw. sind Warenzeichen oder eingetragene Warenzeichen der jeweiligen Inhaber. Die Wiedergabe von Marken, Produktnamen, Gebrauchsnamen, Handelsnamen, Warenbezeichnungen u.s.w. in diesem Werk berechtigt auch ohne besondere Kennzeichnung nicht zu der Annahme, dass solche Namen im Sinne der Warenzeichen- und Markenschutzgesetzgebung als frei zu betrachten wären und daher von jedermann benutzt werden dürften.

Coverbild: www.ingimage.com

Verlag: LAP LAMBERT Academic Publishing GmbH & Co. KG
Heinrich-Böcking-Str. 6-8, 66121 Saarbrücken, Deutschland
Telefon +49 681 3720-310, Telefax +49 681 3720-3109
Email: info@lap-publishing.com

Approved by: Iraq, University of Babylon, Thesis, 2011

Herstellung in Deutschland:
Schaltungsdienst Lange o.H.G., Berlin
Books on Demand GmbH, Norderstedt
Reha GmbH, Saarbrücken
Amazon Distribution GmbH, Leipzig
ISBN: 978-3-8484-2713-0

Imprint (only for USA, GB)
Bibliographic information published by the Deutsche Nationalbibliothek: The Deutsche Nationalbibliothek lists this publication in the Deutsche Nationalbibliografie; detailed bibliographic data are available in the Internet at http://dnb.d-nb.de.
Any brand names and product names mentioned in this book are subject to trademark, brand or patent protection and are trademarks or registered trademarks of their respective holders. The use of brand names, product names, common names, trade names, product descriptions etc. even without a particular marking in this works is in no way to be construed to mean that such names may be regarded as unrestricted in respect of trademark and brand protection legislation and could thus be used by anyone.

Cover image: www.ingimage.com

Publisher: LAP LAMBERT Academic Publishing GmbH & Co. KG
Heinrich-Böcking-Str. 6-8, 66121 Saarbrücken, Germany
Phone +49 681 3720-310, Fax +49 681 3720-3109
Email: info@lap-publishing.com

Printed in the U.S.A.
Printed in the U.K. by (see last page)
ISBN: 978-3-8484-2713-0

Copyright © 2012 by the author and LAP LAMBERT Academic Publishing GmbH & Co. KG and licensors
All rights reserved. Saarbrücken 2012

Spontaneous abortion: Main causes associated with single and recurrent abortion in Iraq

By

Saad M. Al-Aaraji
B.V.M.S., Ph.D
Medical Physiology

Nawras J. Al-Salihi
M.B.Ch.B, M.Sc

Dedication

To…

All Iraqi martyrs who died during violence waves that devastated Iraq in the last few years.

We dedicate this work.

Authors

Acknowledgements

All the praises and thanks are for the most merciful and most compassionate Al-mighty ALLAH, who is entire source of all the knowledge and wisdom to mankind. It is He, who blessed one the courage, ability and sufficient opportunity to complete this task. The authors would like to thank college of medicine, Babylon university and the staff of Physiology department for their support and cooperation.

Best thank and grateful appreciation to Dr. Hadi AL-Mosawi, Department of pathology, for helping in performing the serological and hormonal study of the samples. Our great thanks to Ass. Prof. Dr. Hatem Abdul Lateef ,College of Medicine, for his help in statistical analysis for this work.

We greatly indebted to the medical staff in Emergency department of Gynecology and all members of Medical Laboratories in AL-Hindia General hospital.

Authors

List of Contents

Contents	Page No.
Chapter one /introduction	
1 Introduction	1
1.1 Types of abortion	1
1.1.1 Induced abortion	1
1.1.2 Spontaneous abortion (miscarriage)	1
1.1.2.1 Types of spontaneous abortion (miscarriage)	1
1.1.2.1.1 Threatened abortion	1
1.1.2.1.2 Inevitable abortion	2
1.1.2.1.3 Incomplete abortion	2
1.1.2.1.4 Complete abortion	2
1.1.2.1.5 Missed abortion	2
1.1.2.1.6 Septic abortion	2
1.1.2.1.7 Recurrent abortion	2
1.2 Causes of abortion	2
1.3 The aims of the work	3
Chapter two/ Literatures review	
2. Literature review	4
2.1 Physiological anatomy of female reproductive system	4
2.1.1 Ovaries	5
2.1.2 Fallopian tubes	5
2.1.3 Uterus	5
2.1.4 Vagina	5
2.2 Female Hormonal System	5
2.2.1 Hypothalamic hormone	6
2.2.2 The anterior pituitary hormones	6
2.2.3 Ovarian hormones	7
2.2.3.1 Estrogen hormone	7
2.2.3.2 Progesterone hormone	8
2.2.3.3 Relaxin hormone	9
2.2.3.4 Activins, Inhibins, Follistatin	9
2.3 The Female Monthly Sexual Cycle	9
2.3.1 Follicular phase	10
2.3.2 Ovulation	11
2.3.3 Luteal phase	12
2.4 Pregnancy	12
2.5 Complication of pregnancy	13
2.5.1 Early complication	14
2.5.1.1 Ectopic Pregnancy	14
2.5.1.2 Gestational Trophoplastic Disease (GTD)	14
2.5.1.3 Early Pregnancy Loss (Abortion)	14

2.5.1.3.1 Embryonic losses (early loss)	15
2.5.1.3.2 Fetal losses (late losses)	15
2.6 Types of abortion	15
2.6.1 Induced Abortion	15
2.6.2 Spontaneous Abortion (miscarriage)	16
2.6.2.1 Types of Spontaneous Abortion (miscarriage)	16
2.6.2.1.1 Threatened abortion	16
2.6.2.1.2 Inevitable Abortion	16
2.6.2.1.3 Incomplete Abortion	17
2.6.2.1.4 Complete Abortion	17
2.6.2.1.5 Missed abortion	17
2.6.2.1.6 Septic abortion	17
2.6.2.1.7 Recurrent abortion	18
2.7 Epidemiology of abortion	18
2.8 Causes of abortion	18
2.8.1 Anatomical conditions	19
2.8.1.1 Uterine conditions	19
2.8.1.2 Cervical conditions	20
2.8.2 Genetic disorders	20
2.8.3 Endocrine disorders	21
2.8.3.1 Thyroid disorders	21
2.8.3.2 Diabetes Mellitus	22
2.8.3.3 Poly cystic ovariane syndrome.(PCOS)	23
2.8.3.4 Luteal phase defect(LPD)	23
2.8.4 Thrombophilia	24
2.8.5 Immune factors	25
2.8.5.1 Antiphospholipid syndrome	25
2.8.5.2 Increased uterine Natural Killer (NK) cells	26
2.8.5.3 Parental HLA sharing	26
2.8.5.4 Alloimmune aspects	26
2.8.5.5 Anti-fetal and other antibodies	26
2.8.5.6 Implantation factors	28
2.8.6 Infections	28
2.8.6.1 Toxoplasma infection	29
2.8.6.2 Cytomegalovirus (CMV)	29
2.8.6.3 Rubella	31
2.8.7 Lifestyle factors	31
2.5.2 Late pregnancy complications	32
2.5.2.1 Placenta previa	32
2.5.2.2 Placental abruption	32
Chapter Three/Materials & Methods	
3.1 Materials	33
3.1.1 Patients	33

3.1.2 Control	33
3.1.3 Chemicals	33
3.1.4 Instruments	34
3.2 Methods	35
3.2.1 Medical history (Questionnaire)	35
3.2.2 Blood Collection	35
3.2.3 Biochemical study	35
3.2.3.1 Estimation of fasting blood sugar (FBS)	36
3.2.5 Hematological studies	36
3.2.5.1 Determination of packed cells volume (PCV)	36
3.2.5.2 Estimation of hemoglobin concentration (Hb)	36
3.2.6 Serological study	36
3.2.6.1 Detection of anti-toxoplasmosis (IgM &IgG) antibody	36
3.2.6.2 Detection of anti-cytomegalovirus (IgM & IgG) antibody	37
3.2.6.3 Detection of anti-Rubella (IgM & IgG) antibody	37
3.2.6.4 Detection of antiphospholipid (IgM & IgG)antibody	37
3.2.6.5 Detection of anticardiolipin (IgM & IgG) antibody	37
3.3 Statistical analysis	37
Chapter Four/ Results	
4.1 History of the patients	38
4.1.1 Age distribution in patients with abortion	38
4.1.2 The distribution of patients with single & recurrent abortions according to age groups	38
4.1.3 Age distribution in patients with single & recurrent abortions according to the time of abortion (first and second trimesters of abortions)	40
4.1.4 Age distribution in patients with single abortion according to the time of abortion (first and second trimester of abortions)	40
4.1.5 Age distribution in patients with recurrent abortions according to the time of abortion (first and second trimesters abortions)	41
4.1.6 Family history of abortion	42
4.1.7 Smoking prevalence in abortion	43
4.1.8 Rh-compatability prevalence in abortion	43
4.1.9 History of infertility	44
4.1.10 Abortion and hypertension	44
4.1.11 Abortion & diabetes mellitus	45
4.1.12 Poly cystic ovarian syndrome (PCOs)	46
4.1.13 Anomalies of the female genital tract	47
4.1.14 Abortion and cervical incompetence	47
4.2 Laboratory investigation	47
4.2.1 Packed cell volume (PCV) count	47
4.2.2 Hemoglobin (Hb) concentrations	48

4.2.3 Toxoplasmosis and its relation to abortion	49
4.2.3.1 The distribution of *Toxoplasma gondii* according to the number of patients	49
4.2.3.2 The distribution of *Toxoplasma gondii* according to the ages	50
4.2.3.3 The distribution of *Toxoplasma gondii* according to the trimester of pregnancy	50
4.2.3.4 The distribution of *Toxoplasma gondii* according to the types of antibodies (IgM,IgG)	51
4.2.4 Cytomegalovirus infection and its relation to abortion	52
4.2.4.1 The distribution of CMV infection according to the number of patients	52
4.2.4.2 The distribution of CMV infection according to the ages	53
4.2.4.3 The distribution of CMV infection according to the trimester of pregnancy	53
4.2.4.4 The distribution of CMV infection according to the types of antibodies (IgM, IgG)	54
4.2.5 Rubella infection and its relation to abortion	54
4.2.6 Antiphospholipid antibodies and its relation with abortion	54
4.2 7 Anticardiolipin antibodies and its effect on abortion	55
Chapter Five /Discussion	
5.1 History of the patients	58
5.1.1 Age distribution in patients with abortion	58
5. 1.2 The distribution of patients with single & recurrent abortions according to age groups	58
4.1.3 Age distribution in patients with single & recurrent abortions according to the time of abortion (first and second trimester's abortions)	59
5.1.6 Family history of abortion	59
5.1.7 Smoking prevalence in abortion	60
5.1.8 Rh-incompatability prevalence in abortion	60
5.1.9 History of infertility	61
5.1.10 Abortion and hypertension	61
5.1.11 Abortion & diabetes mellitus	62
5.1.13 Poly cystic ovarian syndrome (PCOs)	62
5.1.14 Anomalies of the female genital tract	62
5.1. 15 Abortion and cervical incompetence	63
5.2 laboratory investigation	63
5.2.1 Packed Cell Volume (PCV) count and Hemoglobin (Hb) concentrations	63
5.2.3Toxoplasmosis and its relation to abortion	64
5.2.3.1 The distribution of *Toxoplasma gondii* according to the number of patients	64
5.2.3.2 The distribution of *Toxoplasma gondii* according to the ages	64

5.2.3.3 The distribution of *Toxoplasma gondii* according to the trimester of pregnancy	65
5.2.3.4 The distribution of *Toxoplasma gondii* according to the type of antibodies	66
5.2.4 Cytomegalovirus (CMV) infection and its relation to abortion	66
5.2.4.1 The distribution of CMV infection according to the number of patients	66
5.2.4.2 The distribution of CMV infection according to the ages	67
5.2.4.3 The distribution of CMV infection according to the trimester of pregnancy	67
5.2.4.4 The distribution of CMV infection according to the type of antibodies	67
5.2.5 Rubella infection and its relation to abortion	68
5.2.6 Antiphospholipid antibodies and its relation with abortion	68
5.2.7 Anticardiolipin antibodies and its effect on abortion	69
Conclusions & Recommendations	
Conclusions	70
Recommendations	71
References	72
Appendices	

Chapter one: Introduction

1 Introduction

Abortion is defined as termination of pregnancy resulting in expulsion of an immature fetus. A fetus of less than twenty week's gestation or a fetus weighing less than 500 gm is considered an abortus (Chan & Johnson, 2006).

Abortion is the most common complication of human gestation, occurring in at least 75% of all women trying to become pregnant, and most of these losses are unrecognized and occur before or during the next expected menses (Thomas, 1999). While 15% to 20% of spontaneous abortions diagnosed after clinical recognition of pregnancy (Khan and Heggen, 1998; Jindal, 2007).

1.1 Types of abortion

There are two types of abortion, the induced abortion and spontaneous abortion (miscarriage).

1.1.1 Induced abortion

Induced abortion is the intentional termination of a pregnancy before the fetus can live independently, it may be elective or therapeutic(Finer & Henshaw, 2003).

1.1.2 Spontaneous abortion (miscarriage)

Spontaneous abortion is that type of abortion which is not induced (Hughes *et al.*, 2007).

1.1.2.1 Types of spontaneous abortion (miscarriage)

There are seven types of spontaneous abortion are present which are;

1.1.2.1.1 Threatened abortion

Threatened abortion is defined as vaginal bleeding occurring in the first 20 weeks of pregnancy, without the passage of tissue or rupture of membranes (Chan & Johnson, 2006). Pain may not be a prominent feature of threatened abortion, although lower abdominal dull ache sometime accompanied the bleeding (Hacker *et al.*, 2010).

1.1.2.1.2 Inevitable abortion

In this case the pregnancy is complicated by both vaginal bleeding and cramp like lower abdominal pain, the cervix is partially dilated, contributing to the inevitability of the process (Monga, 2006).

1.1.2.1.3 Incomplete abortion

Incomplete abortion is characterized by cramping, bleeding, passage of tissue, and a dilated internal os with tissue present in the vagina or endocervical canal. Profuse bleeding, orthostatic dizziness, syncope, postural pulse and blood pressure changes may occur (Chan& Johnson, 2006).

1.1.2.1.4 Complete abortion

The complete abortion is diagnosed when complete passage of products of conception has occurred. The uterus is well contracted, and the cervical os may be closed (Kaufman *et al.*, 2007)

1.1.2.1.5 Missed abortion

Missed miscarriage is gestational sac containing a dead embryo/fetus before 20 weeks gestation without clinical symptoms of expulsion (Monga, 2006).

1.1.2.1.6 Septic abortion

Septic abortion is serious uterine infection during or shortly before or after an abortion (Rana *et al.*, 2004).

1.1.2.1.7 Recurrent abortion

Recurrent abortion or recurrent pregnancy loss (RPL) (medically termed habitual abortion) is defines as three or more successive spontaneous abortions (Gracia *et al.*, 2005). However, some authors suggested that even two spontaneous pregnancy losses constitute recurrent miscarriage and deserve evaluation(Mastenbroek *et al.*, 2007).

1.2 Causes of abortion: Miscarriages can occur for many reasons, not all of which can be identified. about 50% of cases have no cause or association found

and are classified as idiopathic (Bricker and Farquharson, 2002). Some of these causes include:
1. Anatomical conditions: which include uterine conditions and cervical conditions.
2. Genetic disorders.
3. Endocrine disorders: like thyroid diseases, diabetes mellitus, poly cystic ovarian syndrome and luteal phase defect.
4. Thrombophilia.
5. Immune factors: like antiphospholipid syndrome, increase uterine natural killer cells, alloimmune aspects and implantation factors.
6- Infections.
7. Lifestyle factors

1.3 The aims of the work

This work is designed to determine the following:-
1. The incidence of many viral and parasitic diseases in Iraqi women who suffering from single and recurrent abortions through detection of presence of *Toxoplama gondii* parasite, Cytomegalovirus and *Rubella* viruses antibodies in their sera.
2. The immunological changes that associated with single and recurrent abortion through detection of presence of antiphospholipid or anticardiolipin antibodies in the sera of aborted women.
3. Fasting blood sugar in order to determine whether the patients had diabetes mellitus which considered as one of the most important cause of abortion.
4. Doing ultrasonagraphy to evaluate if the patients had poly cystic ovaries, any anomalies in their genital tract or if they had incompetent cervix.
5. Measurement the hemoglobin concentrations (Hb) and packed cell volume (PCV).

Chapter Two: Literatures Review
2. Literatures review
2.1 Physiological anatomy of female reproductive system

The main organs of the human female reproductive tract are the ovaries, fallopian tubes, uterus, and vagina (Guyton &Hall, 2006) (figure 2.1), and the main functions of female reproductive system (Scanlon & Sanders, 2006):-

-Produces ova.

-Secretes sex hormones.

-Receives the male spermatazoa during intercourse.

-Protects and nourishes the fertilized egg until it is fully developed.

-Delivers fetus through birth canal.

-Provides nourishment to the baby through milk secreted by mammary glands in the breast.

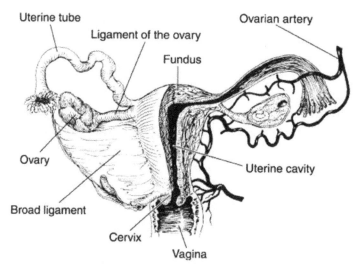

Figure (2.1) The female reproductive system (Guyton & Hall, 2006).

2.1.1 Ovaries

The ovary is an ovum-producing reproductive organ, often found in pairs as part of the female reproductive system (Isachenko *et al.*,2009).

Usually each ovary takes turns releasing eggs every month; however, if there was a case where one ovary was absent or dysfunctional then the other ovary would continue providing eggs to be released (Lan *et al.*, 2008). Ovaries secrete estrogen, progesterone, relaxin ,activins, inhibins, and follistatin hormone (Kimball,2010).

2.1.2 Fallopian tubes

There are two fallopian tubes, also called the uterine tubes or the oviducts. Each fallopian tube attaches to a side of the uterus at one end and at the other end of each fallopian tube is a fringed area that looks like a funnel.

This fringed area, called the infundibulum, lies close to the ovary, but is not attached. Within each tube is a tiny passageway no wider than a sewing needle. When an ovary does ovulate, or release an egg, the egg is swept into the lumen of the fallopian tube by the fimbriae (Scanlon & Sanders, 2006).

2.1.3 Uterus

The uterus is shaped like an upside-down pear, with a thick lining and muscular walls. The uterus contains some of the strongest muscles in the female body. These muscles are able to expand and contract to accommodate a growing fetus and then help push the baby out during labor. These muscles also contract rhythmically during an orgasm in a wave like action. It is thought that this is to help push or guide the sperm up the uterus to the fallopian tubes where fertilization may be possible (Graaff, 2006).

2.1.4 Vagina

The human vagina is an elastic muscular canal that extends from the cervix to the vulva (Jannini *et al.*,2002).

Although there is wide anatomical variation, the length of the un aroused vagina is approximately 6 to 7.5 cm across the anterior wall (front) and 9 cm

(3.5 in) long across the posterior wall (Hines, 2001).

During sexual arousal the vagina expands in both length and width. Its elasticity allows it to stretch during sexual intercourse and during birth (Spence & Melville, 2007).

2.2 Female Hormonal System

The female hormonal system, like that of the male, consists of three hierarchies of hormones; as follows:

2.2.1 Hypothalamic hormone

Gonadotropin-releasing hormone (GnRH), also known as Luteinizing-hormone-releasing hormone (LHRH) and luliberin, is a tropic peptide hormone which synthesized and released from neurons within the hypothalamus so it considered as neurohormone. A key area for production of GnRH is the preoptic area of the hypothalamus, which contains most of the GnRH-secreting neurons. GnRH neurons originate in the nose and migrate into the brain. (Campbell *et al.*, 2009).

At the pituitary gland, GnRH stimulates the synthesis and secretion of the gonadotropins, FSH and LH. These processes are controlled by the size and frequency of GnRH pulses, as well as by feedback from androgens and estrogens. Low-frequency GnRH pulses lead to FSH release, whereas high-frequency GnRH pulses stimulate LH release. The frequency of the pulses varies during the menstrual cycle, and there is a large surge of GnRH just before ovulation (Franceschini *et al.*, 2006).

2.2.2 The anterior pituitary hormones

The anterior pituitary gland secret follicle-stimulating hormone (FSH) and luteinizing hormone (LH), the secretion of these hormones is controlled by pulses of gonadotropin-releasing hormone (GnRH). Those pulses, in turn, are subject to the oestrogen feed-back from the gonads (Fowler *et al.*, 2003).

FSH intiates granulosa cell proliferation and differentiation, antral follicle development, estrogen production, induction of LH receptors on the dominant follicle and inhibin synthesis (Homburg, 2008).

The levels of FSH decline in the late follicular phase, and at the end of the luteal phase, there is a slight rise in FSH that seems to be of importance to start the next ovulatory cycle (DiPiro, 2007) **(figure 2.2)**.

While the level of LH during the early and mid-follicular phase is relatively quiet with pulses every 60-90 minutes and a fairly constant low concentration of circulating LH. However, this is the calm before the storm. An enormous climax is reached with the onset of the LH surge in the late follicular phase the central event of the ovulatory cycle (Homburg, 2008).

This 'LH surge' triggers ovulation thereby not only releasing the egg, but also initiating the conversion of the residual follicle into a corpus luteum that, in turn, produces progesterone to prepare the endometrium for a possible implantation. LH is necessary to maintain luteal function for the first two weeks (Nielsen *et al.*, 2001).

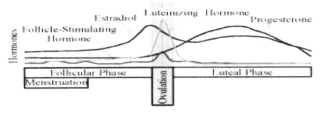

Figure (2.2) Levels of FSH and LH during the female monthly sexual cycle (Nielsen *et al.*, 2001).

2.2.3 Ovarian hormones

The ovaries secret many types of hormones estrogen , progesterone, relaxin ,activins, inhibins and follistatin (Kimball, 2010).

2.2.3.1 Estrogen hormone

The three major naturally occurring estrogens in women are estrone (E1), estradiol (E2), and estriol (E3). Estradiol (E2) is the predominant form in nonpregnant females, estrone is produced during menopause, and estriol is the primary estrogen of pregnancy (Mechoulam *et al.,* 2005).

Estrogen responsible for the conversion of girls into sexually-mature women, it cause broadening of the pelvis, development of breasts, growth of pubic and axillary hair, further development of the uterus and vagina, and increase in adipose (fat) tissue. It is also participate in the monthly preparation of the body for a possible pregnancy and participate in pregnancy if it occurs (Isachenko *et al.*, 2009; Kimball, 2010).

2.2.3.2 Progesterone hormone

Progesterone is steroid hormone that synthesized from pregnenolone which in turn is derived from cholesterol (Schindler *et al.*, 2003).

It produced in the ovaries (to be specific, after ovulation in the corpus luteum), the adrenal glands (near the kidney), and, during pregnancy, in the placenta (Dewick, 2002).

An additional source of progesterone is milk products. They contain much progesterone because on dairy farms cows are milked during pregnancy, when the progesterone content of the milk is high. After consumption of milk products the level of bioavailable progesterone goes up (Goodson *et al.,* 2007).

Progesterone involved in the female menstrual cycle, pregnancy (supports gestation) and embryogenesis of humans, its levels are relatively low during the preovulatory phase of the menstrual cycle, rise after ovulation, and are elevated during the luteal phase(Zarutskiea & Phillips ,2007 ; Cardiol,2009).

It has been observed in animal models that females have reduced susceptibility to traumatic brain injury and this protective effect has been hypothesized to be caused by increased circulating levels of estrogen and progesterone in females (Roof & Hall, 2000).

A number of additional animal studies have confirmed that progesterone has neuroprotective effects when administered shortly after traumatic brain injury (Gibson *et al.*,2008) and encouraging results have also been reported in human clinical trials (Wright *et al.*,2007 ; Xiao *et al.*,2008).The mechanism of progesterone protective effects may be the reduction of inflammation that follows brain trauma(Pan *et al*., 2007).

2.2.3.3 Relaxin hormone

Relaxin is a polypeptide hormone that is produced by the corpus luteum of the ovary, the breast and, during pregnancy, also by the placenta, chorion, and decidua(Becker & Hewitson ,2001).

It rises to a peak within approximately 14 days of ovulation and then declines in the absence of pregnancy resulting in menstruation (Mookerjee *et al*., 2006).

During the first trimester of pregnancy, levels of relaxin rise where additional relaxin is produced by the decidua. Relaxin relaxes the pubic symphysis and other pelvic joints, softens and dilates the uterine cervix. Thus, it facilitates delivery (Wilkinson *et al.*, 2005).

2.2.3.4 Activins, Inhibins, Follistatin

Activin and inhibin are two closely related protein complexes that have opposing biological effects (Chen *et al.*, 2006). Activin enhances FSH biosynthesis and secretion, and participates in the regulation of the menstrual cycle (Sulyok *et al.*, 2004).

Conversely inhibin down regulates FSH synthesis and secretion (van Zonneveld *et al*., 2003). These proteins are synthesized within the follicle and bind to follistatin(Kimball, 2010).

2.3 The female monthly sexual cycle

The normal reproductive years of the female are characterized by monthly rhythmical changes in the rates of secretion of the female hormones and corresponding physical changes in the ovaries and other sexual organs. This rhythmical pattern is called the female monthly sexual cycle (or less accurately, the menstrual cycle) (Guyton & Hall, 2006).

Blood and tissues from the inner lining of the uterus (the endometrium) combine to form the menstrual flow, which generally lasts from 4-7 days. The first period is called menarche. During menstruation arteries that supply the lining of the uterus constrict and capillaries weaken. Blood spilling from the damaged vessels detaches layers of the lining, not all at once but in random patches. Endometrium mucus and blood descending from the uterus, through the liquid creates the menstruation flow (Scanlon & Sanders, 2006).

There are five hormones involved in controlling the female monthly sexual cycle, these are gonadotropin releasing hormone (GnRH) secreted by the hypothalamus, follicle-stimulating hormone (FSH) and lutenizing hormone (LH) secreted by the pituitary gland, and estrogen and progesterone secreted by the ovaries (Carter &Frank, 1986).

Menstrual cycle is commonly divided into three phases: the follicular phase, ovulation, and the luteal phase; although some sources use a different set of phases: menstruation, proliferative phase, and secretory phase (Greenberg *et al.,* 2007) (Figure 2. 3).

The length of each phase varies from woman to woman and cycle to cycle, though the average menstrual cycle is 28 days (Losos *et al.,* 2002).

For an individual woman, the follicular phase often varies in length from cycle to cycle; by contrast, the length of her luteal phase will be fairly consistent from cycle to cycle (Weschler, 2002).

2.3.1 Follicular phase

This phase is also called the proliferative phase because the hormones of this phase causes the lining of the uterus to grow, or proliferate, during this time (Losos *et al.*, 2002).

Through the influence of a rise in follicle stimulating hormone (FSH) during the first days of the cycle, a few ovarian follicles are stimulated ,these follicles, which were present at birth and have been developing for the better part of a year in a process known as folliculogenesis, compete with each other for dominance. When the follicle matures and reaches 8-10 mm in diameter it starts to secrete significant amounts of estradiol (Walter, 2003).

The estrogens initiate the formation of a new layer of endometrium in the uterus. The estrogen also stimulates crypts in the cervix to produce fertile cervical mucus (Weschler, 2002).

Estrogens also suppress production of (LH) from the anterior pituitary gland. When the egg has nearly matured, levels of estradiol reach a threshold above which they stimulate production of LH. These opposite responses of LH to estradiol may be enabled by the presence of two different estrogen receptors in the hypothalamus: estrogen receptor alpha, which is responsible for the negative feedback estradiol-LH loop, and estrogen receptor beta, which is responsible for the positive estradiol-LH relationship (Hu *et al.*, 2008).

2.3.2 Ovulation

Ovulation refers to the release of a viable oocyte from the ovary. The major players in ovulation are gonadotropin releasing-hormone (GnRH), FSH, LH, estrogen and progesterone but essential fine-tuning is provided by a large number of other factors including inhibin, activin and growth factors (Homburg, 2008).

Shortly before ovulation, the protruding outer wall of the follicle swells rapidly, and a small area in the center of the follicular capsule, called the stigma, protrudes like a nipple (Guyton & Hall, 2006).

By the effect of LH, proteolytic enzymes are secreted by the follicle that degrades the follicular tissue at the site of the blister, forming a hole called the stigma. The cumulus-oocyte complex (COC) leaves the ruptured follicle and moves out into the peritoneal cavity through the stigma, where it is caught by the fimbriae at the end of the fallopian tube ((Roberts *et al.*, 2004).

The few days near ovulation constitute the fertile phase. The average time of ovulation is the fourteenth day of an average length (twenty-eight day) menstrual cycle (Susan *et al.*, 2004).

2.3.3 Luteal phase

The second half of the cycle is called the secretory phase in the uterus and the luteal phase in the ovaries (Carter&Frank, 1986; Losos *et al.,* 2002).

Without the ovum, and under the effect of FSH and LH hormones of the pituitary gland ,the follicle folds inward on itself, transforming into the corpus luteum, a steroidogenic cluster of cells that produces estrogen and progesterone(Navarrete-Palacios *et al.*,2003).

These hormones induce the endometrial glands to begin production of the proliferative endometrium and later into secretory endometrium, the site of embryonic growth if fertilization occurs (Susan *et al.*, 2004).

Progesterone plays a vital role in making the endometrium receptive to implantation of the blastocyst and supportive of the early pregnancy. Falling levels of progesterone trigger menstruation and the beginning of the next cycle. From the time of ovulation until progesterone withdrawal has caused menstruation to begin, the process typically takes about two weeks, with ten to sixteen days considered normal (Weschler, 2002).

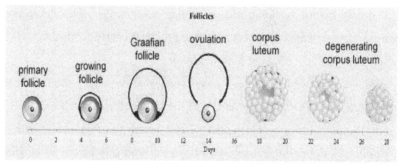

Figure (2. 3) phases of female sexual cycle (Stein Carter, 2004).

2.4 Pregnancy

The pregnancy is sequence of events that are take place in the mother's body when the ovum become fertilized, and the fertilized ovum eventually develops into a full-term fetus (Gyuton & Hall,2006).

Fertilization of the ovum by the sperm usually occurs in the ampulla of the uterine tube. Millions of sperms are deposited in the vagina during intercourse. And only one sperm will success in fertilize the ova (Stovall & Thomas, 2004). After the egg is fertilized by a sperm and then implanted in the lining of the uterus, it develops into the placenta and embryo, and later into a fetus (Iams *et al.*, 2008).

Pregnancy is typically broken into three periods, or trimesters, each of about three months. While there are no hard and fast rules, these distinctions are useful in describing the changes that take place over time (Qasim *et al.*, 1996).

In the first trimester (the first three months) of pregnancy, or the first 13 weeks of pregnancy most organogenesis (development of body organs) occurs (Tracy, 2005).

In the second trimester (the second three months) or weeks 13 to 28 of the pregnancy. Most women feel more energized in this period, and begin to put on weight as the symptoms of morning sickness subside and then fade away, in this period growth occurs and the baby is very active, eventually these movements can be felt by the mother (Prechtl & Heinz, 2007).

The third trimester (the last three months) is a time of rapid growth gaining up to 28 g per day. The baby tends to move less just because the uterus has become so crowded (Dimitrova *et al.,* 2007).

The actual pregnancy duration is typically 38 weeks after conception. Though pregnancy begins at conception, it is more convenient to date from the first day of a woman's last menstrual period, or from the date of conception if known. Starting from one of these dates, the expected date of delivery can be calculated (Norwitz &Errol, 2007).

2.5 Complications of pregnancy

There are two types of complications that are take place during pregnancy; the early complication & the late complications:

2.5.1 Early complications

There are multiple complications that occur early in the pregnancy such as;

2.5.1.1 Ectopic pregnancy

An ectopic pregnancy, or eccyesis, is a complication of pregnancy in which the pregnancy implants outside the uterine cavity. Most ectopic pregnancies (98%) occur in the fallopian tube (so-called tubal pregnancies), but implantation can also occur in the cervix, ovaries, and abdomen and its percentage is about 2% (Shaw *et al.*, 2010).

2.5.1.2 Gestational trophoplastic disease (GTD)

Gestational trophoblastic disease is any type of abnormal proliferation of trophoblasts during pregnancy (Abrão *et al.*, 2007).

The main categories of GTD are complete hydatidiform mole, partial hydatidiform mole and choriocarcenoma (Monga, 2006).

Although the cause of GTD is unknown, it is known to occur more frequently in women younger than 20 years and older than 40 years. Diet may play a causative role, some authors show that molar pregnancy occur at high incidence in geographical area where people consume less β-carotene and folic acid (Hacker *et al*, 2010).

2.5.1.3 Early pregnancy loss (Abortion)

Abortion is defined as termination of pregnancy resulting in expulsion of an immature, nonviable fetus. A fetus of less than twenty week's gestation or a fetus weighing less than 500 gm is considered an abortus (Chan& Johnson, 2006).

Early pregnancy loss is the most common complication of human gestation, occurring in at least 75% of all women trying to become pregnant, and most of these losses are unrecognized and occur before or during the next expected menses (Thomas, 1999).

While 15% to 20% of spontaneous abortions diagnosed after clinical recognition of pregnancy (Khan& Heggen, 1998; Jindal, 2007).

Abortion is considered as nature's method to select for genetically normal offspring (Delhanty *et al.*, 1997).

Many studies showed positive correlation between the number of previous miscarriages and the miscarriage rate in the next pregnancy, as up to 40% of women with three abortions and 50% of women with four abortions will expect fetal loss in their coming pregnancy (Bricker & Farquharson, 2002).

One sporadic abortion generally does not increase the risk of repeated abortion, only about 1% of women have recurrent abortions on two or more than two occasions (Jindal, 2007).

Some authors divided abortion according to the age of the embryo or fetus into; embryonic losses (early loss), and fetal losses (late losses).

2.5.1.3.1 Embryonic losses (early loss)

Embryonic losses (early loss) occur before the 9th gestational week (Potts *et al.*, 1997; Kutteh, 2006), it occur before the full development of baby and are associated with genetic abnormalities in the baby. This type of abortion is generally associated with a small or delayed appearance of gestational sac in ultrasound, empty gestational sac or non- appearance of cardiac pulse (Jindal, 2007).

2.5.1.3.2 Fetal losses (late losses)

Fetal losses (late losses) occur at or after the 9th gestational week to 20th weeks (Potts *et al*, 1997; Kutteh, 2006). The fetal losses is more commonly occur due to many factors like abnormalities in the uterus or immunological factors ,infection and others (Jindal,2007).

2.6 Types of abortion

There are tow types of abortion: The induced abortion and spontaneous abortion (miscarriage);

2.6.1 Induced Abortion

Induced abortion is the intentional termination of a pregnancy before the fetus can live independently.

An abortion may be elective (based on a woman's personal choice) or therapeutic (to preserve the health or save the life of a pregnant woman). (Finer & Henshaw, 2003; Sharp & corp, 2009).

2.6.2 Spontaneous Abortion (miscarriage)

Spontaneous abortion is that type of abortion which is not induced (Sharp &Corp, 2009).

2.6.2.1 Types of Spontaneous Abortion (miscarriage)

There are seven types of spontaneous abortion which are;

-Threatened abortion.

-Inevitable abortion.

-Incomplete abortion.

-Complete abortion.

-Missed abortion.

-Septic abortion.

-Recurrent abortion.

2.6.2.1.1 Threatened abortion

Threatened abortion is defined as vaginal bleeding occurring in the first 20 weeks of pregnancy, without the passage of tissue or rupture of membranes (Chan& Johnson, 2006).

Pain may not be a prominent feature of threatened abortion, although lower abdominal dull ache sometime accompanied the bleeding (Hacker *et al.*, 2010).

According to Monga (2006) one-quarter of all pregnancies are complicated by threatened miscarriage, although many patients may be unaware of their pregnancy when they present with vaginal bleeding.

2.6.2.1.2 Inevitable abortion

In this case the pregnancy is complicated by both vaginal bleeding and cramp like lower abdominal pain, the cervix is partially dilated, contributing to the inevitability of the process (Hacker *et al.*, 2010).

An inevitable abortion can be complete or incomplete, depending on whether or not all fetal and placental tissue has been expelled from the uterus (Monga, 2006).

2.6.2.1.3 Incomplete abortion

Incomplete abortion is characterized by cramping, bleeding, passage of tissue, and a dilated internal os with tissue present in the vagina or endocervical canal. Profuse bleeding, orthostatic dizziness, syncope, postural pulse and blood pressure changes may occur (Chan& Johnson, 2006).

2.6.2.1.4 Complete abortion

The complete abortion is diagnosed when complete passage of products of conception has occurred. The uterus is well contracted, and the cervical os may be closed (Kaufman *et al.*, 2007).

2.6.2.1.5 Missed abortion

Missed miscarriage is gestational sac containing a dead embryo/fetus before 20 weeks' gestation without clinical symptoms of expulsion (Everett, 1997).

When the gestational sac is more than 25 mm in diameter and no embryonic /fetal parts can be seen, the term "blighted ovum" and "an embryonic pregnancy" are used by obstetricians suggesting wrongly that the sac may be develop without an embryo, the explanation for this feature is the early death of an embryo and resorption of the embryo with persistence of the placental tissue rather than a pregnancy originally without an embryo(Monga, 2006).

It is typically caused by a random chromosomal abnormality and accounts for up to 50% of all miscarriage (Chan-Ortega, 2007).

Missed abortion should be suspected when the pregnant uterus fails to grow as expected or when fetal heart tones disappear (Chan& Johnson, 2006).

2.6.2.1.6 Septic abortion

Septic abortion is an infection of the uterus and its appendages following any abortion especially,illegally performed induced abortions. It is characterized by a rise of temperature to at least 100.4°F, associated with offensive or purulent vaginal discharge and lower abdominal pain and tenderness (Rana *et al.*, 2004).

2.6.2.1.7 Recurrent abortion

Recurrent abortion or recurrent pregnancy loss (RPL) (medically termed habitual abortion) is defines as three or more spontaneous abortions (Gracia *et al.*, 2005). However, some authors suggested that even two spontaneous pregnancy losses constitute recurrent miscarriage and deserve evaluation (Mastenbroek *et al.*, 2007).

In a patient with a history of 2 miscarriages, the subsequent risk of pregnancy loss rises to about 25%, whereas 3 abortions raises the risk of a fourth miscarriage to 33% (Jindal, 2007).

2.7 Epidemiology of abortion

Determining the prevalence of miscarriage is difficult. This is because that many miscarriages happen very early in the pregnancy, before a woman may know she is pregnant. Or treatment of women with miscarriage at home means medical statistics on miscarriage miss many cases (Everett, 1997).

Prospective studies using very sensitive early pregnancy tests have found that 25% of pregnancies are miscarried by the sixth week since the woman's Last Menstrual Period (Wilcox *et al.*, 1999; Wang *et al.*, 2003) while clinical miscarriages (those occurring after the sixth week of woman's Last Menstrual Period) occur in 8% of pregnancies (Wang *et al.,* 2003).

2.8 Causes of abortion

Miscarriages can occur for many reasons, not all of which can be identified. Some of these causes include genetic, uterine or hormonal abnormalities, reproductive tract infections, and tissue rejection (Slama *et al.,* 2005).

According to Stirrat (1990); Bricker and Farquharson (2002); about 50% of cases have no cause or association found and are classified as idiopathic.

2.8.1 Anatomical conditions
2.8.1.1 Uterine conditions

Uterine malformation is considered to cause about 15% of recurrent miscarriages (Christiansen *et al.*, 2005). The complications rates with pregnancy are considerably increased; complications include abortion, prematurity, postpartum hemorrhage, retained placenta, and breech presentation (Muckle *et al.*, 2008).

Recurrent pregnancy losses resulting from a uterine septum, bicornuate uterus, intrauterine adhesions, and fibroids mainly occur in the second trimester of pregnancy (Stenchever *et al.*, 2001).

These anatomic abnormalities can be congenital, including diethylstilbestrol-related abnormalities, or acquired, such as intrauterine adhesions or leiomyoma (Stenchever *et al.*, 2001).

Müllerian anomalies have been found in 8% to 10%. Women with müllerian anomalies might be predisposed to recurrent pregnancy loss because of inadequate vascularity to the developing embryo and placenta, reduced intraluminal volume, or cervical incompetence (Abdella *et al.*, 1993& Patton, 1994).

Asherman's syndrome is an acquired uterine disorder characterized by uterine adhesions leading to menstrual disorders, infertility, and possibly pregnancy loss, here miscarriage may be due to impaired implantation secondary to intrauterine fibrosis and endometrial inflammation (Khan& Heggen, 1998).

There are several hypotheses regarding how fibroids may be associated with recurrent pregnancy loss (RPL|). Depending on the fibroid size and location, it may partially obliterate or alter the contour of the intrauterine cavity. It may also provide a poorly vascularized endometrium for implantation or compromise placental development. Uterine fibroids and polyps may also act like an intrauterine device, causing subacute endometritis, and therefore, impair the migration of sperm, ovum, or embryo (Repord, 2006).

2.8.1.2 Cervical conditions

In the second trimester a weak cervix can become a recurrent problem. Such cervical incompetence leads to premature pregnancy loss resulting in miscarriages or preterm deliveries (Christiansen *et al.*, 2005).

Rarely, it may be congenital following inutero exposure to diethylstilbestrol (DES). However, the majority of cases occur as a result of surgical trauma to the cervix from conization, loop electrosurgical excision procedures, over dilation of the cervix during pregnancy termination, or obstetric lacerations (Reprod, 2006).

2.8.2 Genetic disorders

Genetic anomalies are known to be the single most common cause of recurrent abortion, as 5-7% of couples with recurrent miscarriage have one partner with balanced chromosomal rearrangement mainly reciprocal translocations (Simpson & Bombard, 1987).

Almost 40-50% of all early losses are due to genetic abnormalities in the baby. These pregnancies are terminated by nature itself as a defense mechanism against the birth of abnormal babies. Chromosomal investigation of the couple may reveal abnormalities (only in 2-3 % of couple) in any of the parent (Jindal, 2007 ; Alaraji,2010).

The incidence of fetal chromosomal abnormalities is gradually decreasing with duration of pregnancy to less than 1% among live-born children (Stephenson *et al.*, 2002)

It can be argued that most pregnancy losses occur at a preclinical stage and that most of them are due to a genetic abnormality. This hypothesis has, in fact, been corroborated by the data collected by Wilcox *et al.*(1988) they investigated the overall incidence of abortion by measuring daily urinary concentrations of human chorionic gonadotropin (hCG) during menstrual cycles.

With an hCG level above 0.025 ng/mL on 3 consecutive days as a criterion of early pregnancy, they found that 22% of pregnancies ended before pregnancy was clinically detected, and the clinically recognized loss rate was 12% (Dhont, 2003).

Age and success of previous pregnancies are two independent risk factors that affect the loss rate. Many authors have observed an increasing risk of fetal death, in particular spontaneous abortion, with increasing maternal age. The association of age of the mother and the increased likelihood of chromosomal abnormalities is manifested by the age related increase of trisomy 21 and cytogenetic studies on preimplantation embryos (Snijders *et al.*,1999).

In order of frequency, the main chromosomal abnormalities are autosomal trisomies, polyploidy, and monosomy X (Lanasa *et al.*,2001).

2.8.3 Endocrine disorders

The role of endocrine factors in recurrent abortion is controversial, but they are known to contribute to infertility (Khan & Heggen ,1998).

The most common three endocrine disorders that are associated with recurrent pregnancy loss are;

2.8.3.1 Thyroid disorders

In the 1950s and 1960s, hypothyroidism was thought to cause infertility and increased fetal loss (Pratt *et al.*,1993).

However, recent studies that were performed by Pratt *et al.*(1993); Stenchever *et al.*(2001) using radioimmunoassay techniques to assess thyroid function found no evidence that thyroid disease can cause repeated pregnancy loss, and extensive thyroid testing is not warranted nonetheless, measurement of thyroid antibodies can be useful in diagnosing the source of recurrent abortion (Pratt *et al.*,1993).

While the studies which was performed by Grossman *et al.*, 1996; Christiansen *et al.*, 2005; Rao *et al.*, 2008 demonstrated that both hypo- and hyperactivity of thyroid gland increase the risk for pregnancy losses.

Pregnancy complicated with poorly controlled hyperthyroidism is associated with increase rate of spontaneous abortion, preterm delivery, IUGR, stillbirth, preeclampsia, congestive heart failure(Albalovich *et al.*, 2002).

Autoimmune thyroid disease is common in pregnancy. The thyroid peroxidase antibodies (TPA) or antibodies against thyreoglubin are associated with a significant increase in miscarriage rate (Albalovich *et al.*, 2002; Lee *et al.*, 2009).

2.8.3.2 Diabetes Mellitus

Diabetes in pregnant women may be pregestational, where the diabetes (type 1 or type 2) was diagnosed before pregnancy, or gestational, which refers to diabetes diagnosed during pregnancy (Lawrence *et al.*, 2005).

The severity and the duration of type 1 disease and the presence of vascular complications were associated with prematurity and perinatal mortality, whereas for women with type 2 diabetes, poor metabolic control and its consequences were the primary factors associated with adverse perinatal outcome (eg, malformation, macrosomia) (Gonzalez-Gonzalez *et al.*, 2008).

Pre-pregnancy evaluation and counseling of women with pregestational diabetes mellitus (type 1 or type 2) is critical to minimize the risk to the fetus and mother. Women who are in poor glycemic control during the period of fetal organogenesis, which is nearly complete by seven weeks postconception, have a high incidence of spontaneous abortion and fetuses with congenital anomalies (Temple *et al.*, 2002). Thus, the importance of evaluating glycemic control in women with diabetes mellitus and achieving good glycemic control before conception cannot be overstated.

In addition to fetal complications, the physiological changes associated with pregnancy can adversely impact maternal health. Retinopathy, nephropathy, hypertension, neuropathy, cardiovascular disease, and thyroid disease can all affect and be affected by pregnancy (Persson *et al.*, 2009).

According to the study that is performed by Alexander *et al.* (1983) on a group of pregnant women complaining from insulin dependent diabetic mellitus, they found that the level of glycosylated haemoglobin (HbA1C) which reflects overall blood glucose control over the previous 2 months, was abnormally high and eventually their pregnancy was complicated by spontaneous abortion, also it associated with a greater prevalence of major congenital anomalies in the infants (Mill *et al.*, 1988).

2.8.3.3 Poly cystic ovariane syndrome.(PCOS)

Patients with PCOs appear to have an increased risk of spontaneous abortion. This has been attributed to hyperinsulinemia that increases pulse activity of GnRH leading to disorderly LH and FSH activity (Dungan *et al*., 2006) .Elevated levels of luteinising hormone (LH) may produce an adverse environment for the oocyte, perhaps even inducing premature maturation and completion of the first meiotic division (Regan *et al.*, 1989; Khan & Heggen ,1998 ; Rai *et al* .,2000).

More recently, the focus has been shifted to insulin resistance or excess androgens as a possible explanation for the increased incidence of abortion in patients with PCOS (Wang *et al.*, 2002; Christiansen *et al.*, 2005).

Lastly and according to the study that performed by Khattab *et al.*(2006) it have been found that administration of metformin throughout pregnancy to women with PCOS was associated with a marked and significant reduction in the rate of early pregnancy loss .

2.8.3.4 Luteal phase defect (LPD)

Luteal phase defect is defined as a deficiency in the amount and/or duration of steroidogenesis, and is characterized by inadequate endometrial maturation (Khan & Heggen ,1998 ; Bulletin , 2001).

Oligomenorrhoea has been shown to be an independent adverse risk factor for pregnancy loss in a recurrent pregnancy loss population and this group of women has lower luteal phase estradiol levels suggesting poor endometrial receptivity (Bricker & Farquharson, 2002).

Although luteal phase defects have long been a paradigm of an endocrine cause of infertility and early pregnancy wastage, the definition, diagnosis, and, hence, the relation to infertility in general are still very confusing. Initially, a distinction was made between a short luteal phase and a deficient luteal phase. Particularly the latter was deemed to be associated with early pregnancy wastage (Dhont, 2003).

The condition can be diagnosed by serial serum progesterone estimations, endometrial biobsy, also it can be diagnosed by ultrasonographic measurement of endometrial thickness, and/or endometrial protein analysis (Khan & Heggen, 1998).

Treatment of LPD is controversial due to a lack of controlled studies. The most popular therapy is progesterone supplementation, either by vaginal suppository or intramuscular injection. Other options include clomephene citrate and supportive doses of human chorionic gonadotrophins (hCG) during the luteal phase. The reported pregnancy success rate with treatment is 70% to 80% (Pratt *et al.*, 1993).

While according to the study of Nardo *et al.* (2002) there is no solid evidence for a beneficial effect of supplementation of the luteal phase with either progesterone or hCG. This is not surprising, because the origin of luteal-phase deficiency could as well originate in the preceding follicular phase, making the endometrium unresponsive to an extraprogestational or a luteotrophic stimulus.

2.8.4 Thrombophilia

Thrombophilia is hypercoagulability state in which the vascularity of the placenta is affected these abnormalities of placental vasculature may result in a number of gestational pathologies, including first- and second-trimester miscarriages, intrauterine growth restriction (IUGR), intrauterine fetal death, placental abruption and pre-eclampsia (Bianca *et al.*, 2010).

The most common problem in hereditary thrombophilia is the factor V Leiden and prothrombin mutation (Wramsby *et al*.,2000; Bulletin,2001 ;Christiansen *et al.*, 2005).

Thrombophilia may explain up to 15% of recurrent miscarriages (Christiansen *et al.*, 2005). Some preliminary studies suggest that anticoagulant medication may improve the chances of carrying pregnancy to term but these studies need to be confirmed before they are adopted in clinical practice (Rodger , 2008).

2.8.5 Immune factors
2.8.5.1 Antiphospholipid syndrome

Antiphospholipid syndrome (APS or APLS) or antiphospholipid antibody syndrome is a disorder of coagulation that causes blood clots (thrombosis) in both arteries and veins as well as pregnancy-related complications such as miscarriage, stillbirth, preterm delivery, or severe preeclampsia (Pattision *et al.*, 1998 ; Rauch, 1999).

Antiphospholipid syndrome is autoimmune disease, in which antiphospholipid antibodies (Anticardiolipin antibodies and Lupus anticoagulant) react against proteins that bind to anionic phospholipids on plasma membranes(Hughes , 2009).

The term "primary antiphospholipid syndrome" is used when APS occurs in the absence of any other related disease while the term "secondary antiphospholipid syndrome" is used when APS coexists with other diseases such us systemic lupus erythematos. In rare cases, APS leads to rapid organ failure due to generalised thrombosis and a high risk of death; this is termed "catastrophic antiphospholipid syndrome" (CAPS)(Balasch *et al.*, 1996 ; Diejomaoh *et al.,* 2002).

2.8.5.2 Increased uterine Natural Killer (NK) cells

A controversial area is the presence of increased natural killer cells in the uterus. It is poorly understood whether these cells actually inhibit the formation of a placenta, and it has been noted that they might be essential for this process (Rodger, 2008).

A 2004 paper (Moffett *et al*.) warned that determination of NK cells in peripheral blood does not predict uterine NK cell numbers, because they are a different class of lymphocytes, and state that immunosuppressive treatments are not warranted

2.8.5.3 Parental HLA sharing

Two recent studies made by Aldrich *et al*.(2001) & Pfeiffer *et al.* (2001), have shown that the sharing of certain Human leukocyte antigen-G (HLA-G) alleles by both partners was significantly associated with an increased risk for miscarriage.

2.8.5.4 Alloimmune aspects

For several decades it has been speculated that a defect in the maternal immune response to the semiallogeneic fetal graft could be involved in the mechanism of abortion.

In fact, because the fetus is a semiallograft, some protective immunologic mechanisms should be involved to prevent maternal rejection. Paradoxically, opposing parental histocompatibility seems to be necessary for maintaining pregnancy by induction of protective blocking antibodies. This hypothesis makes sense from a teleologic and evolutionary point of view, because it would guarantee reproductive heterogeneity ((Lim *et al.,* 1996 ; Dhont,2003).

2.8.5.5 Anti-fetal and other antibodies

Maternal embryotoxic antibodies, induced by fetal or paternal antigenes, could interfere with fetal survival. A classic example is the late pregnancy loss caused by anti-D antibodies in Rhesus-negative women (Simpson *et al.,* 1996).

Rh incompatibility is a condition that occurs when the mother of a fetus or newborn has Rh-negative blood type and the fetus or newborn has Rh-positive blood. This incompatible blood reaction may cause problems in newborn as well as life-threatening problems for future pregnancies (McLaughlin, 2008).

The build up of antibodies does not usually occur until after delivery of the newborn. However, not all women develop antibodies to the Rh factor after having one baby with Rh-positive blood. Generally, there is no effect on the first-born child. If problems occur, they generally happen in second and later pregnancies (Hannifin, 2006).

The woman who is Rh negative becomes pregnant again and her unborn baby has Rh-positive blood. The Rh antibodies that the woman may have developed during or after her first pregnancy can pass through the blood to her second baby and attack the baby's red blood cells. This attack can cause hemolysis, which is the destruction of red blood cells. The baby may start to produce more red blood cells in an effort to replace the ones that were destroyed (McLaughlin, 2008).

The amount of fetal blood necessary to produce Rh incompatibility varies, in one study, less than 1 mL of Rh-positive blood was shown to sensitize volunteers with Rh-negative blood. Conversely, other studies have suggested that 30% of persons with Rh-negative blood never develop Rh incompatibility, even when challenged with large volumes of Rh-positive blood. Once sensitized, it takes approximately one month for Rh antibodies in the maternal circulation to equilibrate in the fetal circulation. In 90% of cases, sensitization occurs during delivery. Therefore, most firstborn infants with Rh-positive blood type are not affected because the short period from first exposure of Rh-positive fetal erythrocytes to the birth of the infant is insufficient to produce a significant maternal IgG antibody response.

Several studies have shown an increased frequency of antisperm antibodies among women experiencing abortions. Pregnancy could be endangered by cross-reaction with paternally derived antigens, which might be essential for embryonic survival (Branch *et al.*, 2001).

In a large, prospective study, however, Simpson *et al.* (1996) found no difference in the incidence of antisperm antibodies in women who experienced pregnancy loss and controls.

2.8.5.6 Implantation factors

Implantation is a complex and finely programmed process, involving many interactions within and between maternal and fetal cell populations. Polypeptide factors called cytokines supply crucial signals, possibly exerting a positive effect on implantation.

The endometrium is an active producer of cytokines, which may be required for both blastocyst attachment and maternal recognition of pregnancy and communication with the embryo. Hence, a cytokine defect can lead to implantation failure but the exact mechanism for this has not yet been established (Khan &Heggen, 1998).

2.8.6 Infections

A number of maternal infections can lead to a single pregnancy loss, including listeriosis, toxoplasmosis, and certain viral infections such as rubella, herpes simplex, measles, cytomegalovirus, coxsackie virus (Christiansen *et al.,* 2005).

Various infectious mechanisms may explain sporadic (but not recurrent) miscarriage including toxic metabolic byproducts, exotoxins, endotoxins, or cytokines (AL-Hamdani & Mahdi, 1997; Khan & Heggen, 1998).

Brucellosis is one of the most common zoonotic diseases that can be encountered during pregnancy; it can be associated with abortion, congenital and neonatal infections and infection of the delivery team (Karcaaltincaba *et al*, 2010).

2.8.6.1 Toxoplasma infection

Toxoplasmosis is a systemic disease caused by the protozoan Toxoplasma gondii. The organism is acquired by ingesting under cooked meat or unpasteurized goat's milk, drinking contaminated water (Singh, 2003), or exposure to feces from an infected cat (Bowie *et al.*, 1997).

Between 15% and 40% of women of reproductive age have antibody (IgG) to Toxoplasma gondii and therefore are immune to future infection. In immunocompromised women such as those with AIDS a reactivation of toxoplasma could occur that would potentially be associated with a risk of fetal infection (Cook *et al.*, 2000).

The risk of transitions to the fetus is 15 % in the first trimester, 25 % in the second trimester and 65 % in the third trimester (Kapperud *et al.*, 1996; Dunn *et al.*, 1999).

The severity of fetal infection is greatest with first-trimester infection, and congenital defects are rarely seen if the infection occurs after 20 weeks of gestation. About 15 % of infants with congenital infection are symptomatic at birth. A classic triad of hydrocephalus, intracranial calcifications, and chorioretinitis is described. Of the asymptomatic infants, 25% to 50% exhibit later sequelae (Hacker *et al.*, 2010)

2.8.6.2 Cytomegalovirus (CMV) infection

Cytomegalovirus (CMV) is the largest member of the herpes virus family, with a double-stranded DNA genome (Schleiss, 2010). CMV in humans it is commonly known as HCMV or Human Herpes virus 5 (HHV-5) (Ryan & Ray, 2004).

All herpes viruses share a characteristic ability to remain latent within the body over long periods(Staras *et al.*, 2006) .Infectious CMV may be shed in the bodily fluids of any infected person, and can be found in urine, saliva, blood, tears, semen, and breast milk. The shedding of virus can occur intermittently, without any detectable signs or symptoms (Caruso *et al.*, 2009).

About half of pregnant women have had CMV in the past and most do not need to be concerned about it during pregnancy. However, an infected woman can pass the virus on to her baby during pregnancy and breastfeeding (Duff, 2007).

Most infected babies have no serious problems from the virus. However, studies suggest that babies are more likely to develop serious complications when their mother is infected in the first 20 weeks of pregnancy (Adler, 2007).

Children with congenital CMV infection following first trimester maternal infection are more likely to have central nervous system (CNS) sequelae, especially sensor neural hearing loss, than are those whose mothers were infected later in pregnancy. However, some degree of CNS impairment can follow even late gestational infection (Robert *et al.*, 2006).

The cause for that and according to the study that performed by Malm & Engman (2007) is that during early pregnancy, CMV has a teratogenic potential and may cause malformations such as migrational disturbances in the brain, which can be visualized using neuroimaging methods such as magnetic resonance imaging (MRI) in such children.

The enzyme-linked immunosorbent assay (or ELISA) is the most commonly available serologic test for measuring antibody to CMV. The result can be used to determine if acute infection, prior infection, or passively acquired maternal antibody in an infant is present. Other tests include various fluorescence assays, indirect hemagglutination, Polymrase chain reaction (PCR) and latex agglutination. If serologic tests detect a positive or high titer of IgG, this result should not automatically be interpreted to mean that active CMV infection is present. However, if antibody tests of paired serum samples show a fourfold rise in IgG antibody and a significant level of IgM antibody, meaning equal to at least 30% of the IgG value, or virus is cultured from a urine or throat specimen, the findings indicate that an active CMV infection is present (Kearns *et al.*, 2002).

2.8.6.3 Rubella infection

Rubella (German measles) is a viral illness caused by a Toga virus of the genus Rubi virus and is characterized by a maculopapular rash (Banatvala & Brown, 2004).

Rubella virus specific IgM antibodies are present in people recently infected by Rubella virus but these antibodies can persist for over a year and a positive test result needs to be interpreted with caution (Best, 2007). The presence of these antibodies along with, or a short time after, the characteristic rash confirms the diagnosis (Stegmann & Carey, 2002). There is no specific treatment for Rubella; however, management is a matter of responding to symptoms to diminish discomfort. (Khandekar *et al.,* 2007).

2.8.7 Lifestyle factors

While lifestyle factors have been associated with increased risk for miscarriage, and are usually not listed as specific causes for RPL, every effort should be made to address these issues in patients with RPL. Of specific concern are chronic exposures to toxins including smoking, alcohol, and drugs (Bulletin, 2001), example of these drugs is Isotretinoin which is a retinoic acid used to treat severe acne and is associated with spontaneous abortion (McGregor, 2000).

Maternal exposure to environmental tobacco smoke for 1 hour or more per day was associated with spontaneous abortion, even. For both maternal direct and environmental exposure, the association appeared to be stronger in second-trimester abortions (Windham *et al.,* 1992).

Heavy metals (such as lead and mercury), organic solvents, and ionizing radiation are confirmed environmental teratogens, and exposure could contribute to pregnancy loss. Hyperthermia is suspected teratogens, while the effect of pesticides remains unknown (Rasch, 2003). For repetitive losses to occur, some chronic exposure to toxic agents should be assumed. Consumption of five or more units of alcohol per week and 375 mg or more caffeine per day during pregnancy was found to increase the risk of spontaneous abortion (Cnattingius *et al.*, 2000; Rasch, 2003).

In 2008, a large cohort study of 1063 patients by Weng *et al.* demonstrated that caffeine consumption had a dose-dependent increase in the risk of miscarriage at all levels of consumption. Patients with caffeine intake of less than 200 mg/d were 1.42 times more likely to have an early miscarriage, whereas in those with intake of 200 mg/d or greater, the risk increased to 2.23 times compared with patients with no caffeine use. In addition, the magnitude of the association appeared to be stronger among women without a history of miscarriage than that among women with such a history.

But some authors doubt the validity of most studies on caffeine intake and the risk of abortion (Leviton & Cowan, 2002). The relative risk of spontaneous abortion from exposure to anesthetic gas was 1.9%(McGregor ,2000)

2.5.2 Late pregnancy complications: There are multiple complications that occur late in the pregnancy such as ;(Francois & Foley, 2007):

2.5.2.1 Placenta previa

Placenta praevia is an obstetric complication in which the placenta is attached to the uterine wall close to or covering the cervix. It can sometimes occur in the later part of the first trimester, but usually during the second or third. It is a leading cause of antepartum haemorrhage (vaginal bleeding). It affects approximately 0.5% of all labours (Bhide & Thilaganathan, 2004).

2.5.2.2 Placental abruption

Placental abruption (also known as abruptio placentae) is one of the complication of pregnancy, where in the placental lining has separated from the uterus of the mother. It is the most common pathological cause of late pregnancy bleeding. It occurs in 1% of pregnancies world wide with a fetal mortality rate of 20–40% depending on the degree of separation. Placental abruption is also a significant contributor to maternal mortality (Usui *et al.*, 2007).

Chapter Three: Materials and Methods
3.1 Materials
3.1.1 Patients

The study lasted from November/2009 to May/2010. In this study eighty seven women who had single or recurrent abortions were included. They were divided into three age groups. The number of each group range from 9 to 49 women .The ages of these groups were divided as follows:

Age group1: $\leq$ 15 to 25 years.

Age group 2: 26 to 35 years.

Age group 3: 36 to 45 years.

The samples were taken from AL-Hindiya General Hospital. All the patients were suffering from single or recurrent abortions and clinically assessed by a gynecologist.

3.1.2 Control

Twenty healthy women were selected randomly as a control group without any history of abortion. They were 15 pregnant women in first and second trimesters of pregnancy and the rest are not pregnant women. They were almost similar to patients in age ranges, occupation, social and economic status and their residence.

The control subjects were consisting of three age groups of healthy subjects without any history of abortion, clinically assessed by a specialist. Each group consists of about 3 to 12 women .Their ages were ranged as follows:

Age group 1: $\leq$ 15 to 25 years.

Age group 2: 26 to 35 years.

Age group 3: 36 to 45 years.

3.1.3 Chemicals

The following table refers to the chemicals materials used in this work and their sources (Table 3.1).

Table 3.1: The chemicals and materials used in this study and their sources.

No.	Chemical Material	Sources
1	Toxoplasma IgG kit by ELISA	BioCheck; Spain
2	Toxoplasma IgM kit by ELISA	BioCheck; Spain
3	Cytomegalovirus IgM kit by ELISA	BioCheck; Spain
4	Cytomegalovirus IgG kit by ELISA	BioCheck; Spain
5	Rubella virus IgG kit by ELFA	BioMerux;France
6	Rubella virus IgM kit by ELFA	BioMerux; France
7	Anticardiolipin IgM antibody assays kit by ELISA	Aeskulisa;Germany
8	Anticardiolipin IgG antibody assays kit by ELISA	Aeskulisa;Germany
9	Antiphospholipid IgM antibody assays kit by ELISA	Aeskulisa;Germany
10	Antiphospholipid IgG antibody assays kit by ELISA	Aeskulisa;Germany
11	Blood glucose kit	Linear chemicals; spain

3.1.4 Instruments

The following table (3.2) refers to the main instruments used in this study.

Table 3.2: The instruments used in this study and their sources.

No.	Instrument	Sources
1	ELISA Reader	Beckman Coulter, Austria
2	Hemocytometer	Osaka , Japan
3	Centrifuge.	Heareus, Germany
4	Spectrophotometer	Optima; Japan
5	Plain tube	AFma – Dispo, Jordan
6	EDTA tube	AFma – Dispo, Jordan
7	Automatic pipette 50,100,500 µl	Germany Slamed
8	Micro – pipette 100 -1000 µl	Oxford ,USA
9	Micro – pipette 50 µl	Oxford ,USA
10	Disposal syringe.	Asia medical instrument roratoional
11	Refrigerator	Concord ,Lebanon
12	Apendroff tubes	Esplf-Germany

3.2 Methods

3.2.1 Medical history (Questionnaire)

A well-structured questionnaire was developed for the study and was filled for every patient and control (Appendix I).

3.2.2 Blood Collection

Five ml of venous blood samples were obtained from antecubital vein of the patient and control groups. The arm should be warm to improve blood circulation and distended the vein. A tourniquet was applied directly on the skin around the arm (usually from the left arm), approximately 6 to 8 cm above the site of collection. The skin over the vein was sterilized with a small pad of cotton wool soaked with 70% ethyl alcohol. Needles used were with 19 to 21 gauges. The site was dried with clean gauze, to prevent hemolysis by alcohol.

The blood sample that obtained from each subjects was divided into two parts, the first part was 3ml of blood that put on plain tubes, to be used for preparing sera for subsequent biochemical and serological tests .while the second part consist of 2ml of blood was put in tubes contain ethylene diamine tetra acetate (EDTA) as anti-coagulants to prevent clotting of blood to be used for hematological studies.

The blood in the plain tubes was allowed to clot for 45 minutes at room temperature, sera were obtained and separated by centrifugation for 15 minutes at 3000 r.b.m. (round per minute) and precautions were taken to avoid hemolysis and the serum obtained was put in ependroff tubes and stored in deep freeze for biochemical tests.

Each sample was labeled and given a serial number together with the patient name, the serum samples were stored at -20°C for biochemical and serological analysis (Lewis *et al.*, 2006).

3.2.3 Biochemical study

In this study the Biochemical test which performed was the fasting blood sugar that measured in the sera of both patients and control groups.

3.2.3.1 Estimation of fasting blood sugar (FBS)

The level of fasting blood sugar (FBS) for patients and control was measured using Enzymatic colorimetric method, the kit that was used was manufactured by Linear chemicals, S.L., Spain.

We adapted test procedure and protocol recommended by the kit manufacturer which was given in details in the kit's leaflet (Appendix).

3.2.4 Hematological studies

3.2.4.1 Determination of packed cells corpuscle

Microhematocrit method was used to determine PCV in which the blood was permitted to fill to approximately three quarters of the capillary tubes lengths then the unmarked end is closed with modeling clay and centrifuged in the microhematocrit centrifuge. After centrifugation for 15 minutes at a speed of 14,500 rpm, the proportion of the RBC (red blood corpuscles) column to the total column (i.e. PCV) was determined by using a special graded circular ruler especially designed for PCV measurement (Lewis *et al.*, 2006).

3.2.4.2 Estimation of hemoglobin concentration (Hb)

A cyanomethemoglobin method was used to estimate the hemoglobin contents of the blood. The method was based on Drabkins cyanide- ferric cyanide solution and a 20 µL of blood was added to 5 ml of Drabkins 's solution, mixing, and incubated for at least 5 minutes at 37°C and then the results were estimated by using hemoglobinmeter at 450 nm wave length (Lewis *et al.*,2006).

3.2.5 Serological study

3.2.5.1 Detection of anti-Toxoplasmosis (IgM &IgG) antibody

The anti Toxoplasma antibodies (IgM and IgG) were detected in the sera of the patients by using ELISA technique the kits which used were ELISA kits from BioCheck Inc. (Spain). The procedure was performed according to manufacture instructions (Appendix).

3.2.5.2 Detection of anti-Cytomegalovirus (IgM & IgG) antibody

The anti cytomegalovirus antibodies (IgM and IgG) were detected in the sera of the patients by using ELISA technique the kits which used were ELISA kits from Biokit Co. (Spain). The procedure was performed according to manufacture instructions (Appendix   ).

3.2.5.3 Detection of anti-Rubella (IgM & IgG) antibody

The level of anti-Rubella (IgM & IgG) antibody for patients and control was measured using Enzymatic Linked Fluorescent Assay (ELFA) technique, the kit that was used was manufactured by BioMerux; France. We adapted test procedure and protocol recommended by the kit manufacturer which was given in details in the kit's leaflet (Appendix   ).

3.2.5.4 Detection of antiphospholipid (IgM & IgG)antibody

The antiphospholipid antibodies (IgM and IgG) were detected in the sera of the patients by using ELISA technique; the kits which used were ELISA kits from Aeskulisa (Germany). The procedure was performed according to manufacture instructions (Appendix   ).

3.2.5.5 Detection of anticardiolipin (IgM & IgG) antibody

The anticardiolipin antibodies (IgM and IgG) were detected in the sera of the patients by using ELISA technique, the kits which used were ELISA kits from Aeskulisa (Germany). The procedure was performed according to manufacture instructions (Appendix   ).

3.3 Statistical analysis

The data were analyzed by using computerized SPSS (Statistical Package of Social Science) program; the analysis of variance (ANOVA) and x^2 test were used to determine the differences between the three groups and within groups. A p value < 0.05 is considered to be statistically significant (Daniel, 1999).

Chapter Four: Results

4.1 History of the patients

A total number of 107 patients were included in this study, 87 had abortion and 20 are control group. Of those 87 patients there were 58 patients had recurrent abortion and 29 patients had single abortion.

4.1.1 Age distribution in patients with abortion

The patients under study were divided according to age in to three age groups the most higher incidence of abortion observed in the ages between ≤ 15 to 25 years age group followed by 26 to 35 years age group (Figure 4-1).

The higher incidence of single abortion was in the age groups between ≤15 to 25 years (63.0%), followed by 29.6% in the ages between 26 to 35 years then the age between 36 to 45 years (7.4%), there is significant differences ($p < 0.05$) between these groups.

While in the recurrent abortions group we found that the higher incidence of abortion (53.4%) occurred in the age groups between 26 to 35 years followed by (39.7%) in the age group between ≤15 to 25 years and then (6.9%) in the age groups between 36 to 45 years, there is significant differences ($p < 0.05$) between the age groups (26 to 35) years and (36 to 45).

In the control group there were 46.7% of the persons their ages range between ≤15 to 25 years, 33.3% their ages range between 26 to 35 years &20.0% of the persons their ages range between 36 to 45 years.

4.1.2 Distribution of patients with single & recurrent abortions according to age groups

In this study we found that recurrent abortions represent the higher incidence in all age groups as we compare it with the single abortion .These incidences were 79.4%,66.6% and 54.75%, in the age groups 26 to 35 years, 36 to 45 years and ≤15 to 25 years respectively.

While in the single abortion group the incidences were 45.2%, 33.3% and 20.42% in the ages≤15 to 25 years, 36 to 45 years and 26 to 35 years respectively.

Chapter Four —————————————————————————— Results

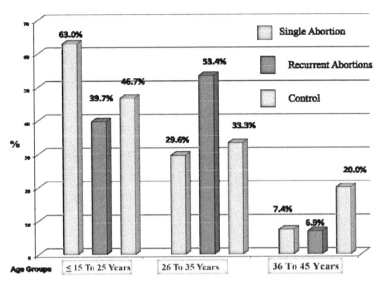

Figure 4.1: Age distribution in patients with abortions and control groups.

When these data analyzed statistically we found that there is significant differences (p <0.05) between single and recurrent abortions regarding the age groups 26 to 35 years and 36 to 45 years (Figure 4.2).

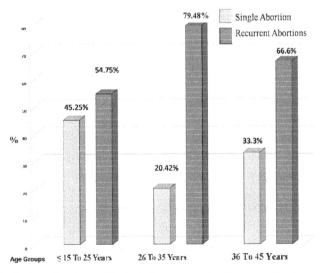

Figure 4.2: Distribution of patients with single & recurrent abortions according to age groups.

4.1.3 Age distribution in patients with single and recurrent abortions according to the time of abortion

Figure (4.3) show that in the age group between ≤15 to 25 years and 26 to 35 years the incidence of abortions that occur in the first trimester of the pregnancy is much higher than the incidence of abortions that occur in the second trimester of the pregnancy which were 71.42 % and 53.58% for first trimester abortions and 28.58% and 46.15% for the second trimester abortions. There is significant differences ($p < 0.05$) between first and second trimesters regarding the age groups ≤15 to 25 years. While the percentage of abortion in the first and second trimester of the pregnancy was equal (50%) in the age group 36 to 45 years ($p > 0.05$).

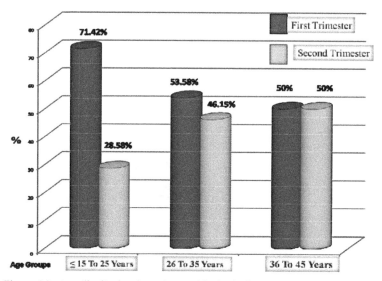

Figure 4.3: Age distribution in patients with single & recurrent abortions according to the time of abortion (first and second trimester's abortions).

4.1.4 Age distribution in patients with single abortion according to the time of abortion (first and second trimester of abortions)

According to results of this study we found that the percentage of first trimester abortion was equal (62.5%) in the age group between ≤ 15 to 25 and

40

26 to 35 years and so there is no significant differences (p>0.05),but there is significant differences (p<0.05) between these two groups and the age group 36 to 45 years were they had incidence (50%) at the same time the age group 36 to 45 years was show high incidence of second trimester abortions (50%) as we compared it with the incidence of second trimester abortions in the age group ≤ 15 to 25 and 26 to 35 years, where they had equal incidence(37%) of second trimester abortions (p<0.05)(Figure 4.4).

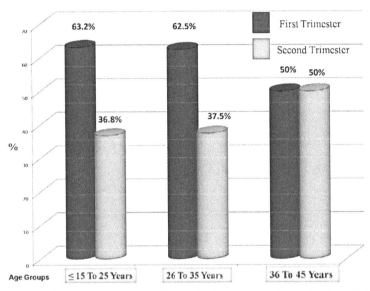

Figure 4.4: Age distribution in patients with single abortion according to the time of abortion (first and second trimester's abortions).

4.1.5 Age distribution in patients with recurrent abortions according to the time of abortion (first and second trimester´s abortions)

As shown in figure (4.5) the higher percentage of first trimester abortions was 78.3% and related to the age group between ≤ 15 to 25 years ,while the age group between 26 to 35 & 36 to 45 years recorded equal percentage of first trimester abortions which was 50% .While the second trimester abortion had lowest value (21.7%) in the age group ≤ 15 to 25 years & (50%) ,(48.4%) in the age group 36 to 45 years, & 26 to 35 years respectively. There is significant differences (p<0.05) between the age group ≤ 15 to 25 years and the other two groups regarding first trimester abortions and second trimester abortions.

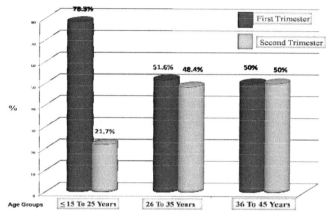

Figure 4.5: Age distribution in recurrent abortions group according to the time of abortion.

4.1.6 Family history of abortions

This study demonstrated that 25.8% of the patients with recurrent abortion had positive family history of abortion while in the single abortion group the percentage of positive family history of abortion was 24.1%. So there is highly significant relationship ($p < 0.01$) between positive family history of abortion and abortions (Figure 4.6).

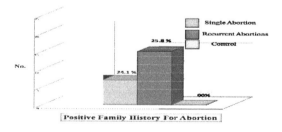

Figure 4.6: Positive family history for abortions in patients who had single, recurrent, single & recurrent abortions and control groups.

4.1.7 Smoking prevalence in abortions

According to patient's history, 20.6% of the patients with recurrent abortions and 17.2% of the patient with single abortion were smoker (figure 4.7). There is significant relationship (P <0.05) between smoking and abortion.

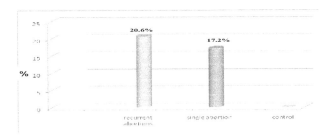

Figure 4.7: Smoking and it's associated with abortions in patients who had single, recurrent, single &recurrent abortions and control groups.

4.1.8 Rh-compatability prevalence in abortion

The figure 4.8 show that there were 3 patients with recurrent abortions who are Rh-incompatable with their husbands which constitute 5.1% and 1 patient with single abortion which constitute 3.4%, there is significant differences (p <0.05) between the patients and control groups.

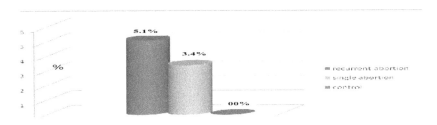

Figure 4.8: Rh-compatability in association with abortions in patients who had single, recurrent, single &recurrent abortions and control groups.

4.1.9 History of infertility

According to the history of the patients, there were 5 patients with single and recurrent abortions had primary infertility which constitute 5.7%,1 of them had single abortion that constitute 3.4% & 4 had recurrent abortions which constitute 6.8%,and also there were 5 patients with single &recurrent abortions had secondary infertility which constitute 5.7% ,2 of them had single abortion which constitute 6.8% &3 of them had recurrent abortions that constitute 5.1%.There is significant differences ($p < 0.05$) between the patients and control groups(Table 4.1).

Table 4.1: Frequency distribution of infertility in patients who had single, recurrent, single &recurrent abortions and control group.

Groups	infertility			
	primary		secondary	
	No.	%	No.	%
Single& recurrent abortions	5	5.7	5	4.6
Single abortion	1	3.4	2	6.8
Recurrent abortions	4	6.8	3	5.1
Control	00	00	00	00

4.1.10 Abortion and hypertension

After taking history of the patients and measuring their blood pressure, results found that in single abortion group there were equal incidence (6.8%) of the development of gestational hypertension in the age group ≤15 to 25 and 26 to 35 years, while there was no case recorded in the age between 36 to 45 years. There were no significant differences ($p > 0.05$) between age groups.

While in the recurrent abortion group, the higher incidence (5.1%) of the development of gestational hypertension was in the ages between ≤15 to 25 years, followed by 3.4% and 1.7% in the ages 26 to 35 and 36 to 45 respectively.

There is significant differences (p<0.05) between the age groups ≤15 to 25 years and the age group 36 to 45 years, also there is significant differences (p < 0.05) between single and recurrent abortion group regarding the age 36 to 45 years . So there is significant relationship (p < 0.05) between abortion and hypertension (Figure 4.9).

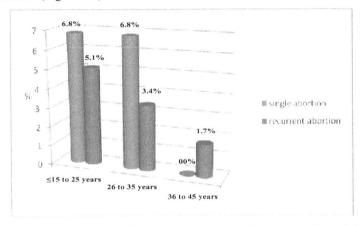

Figure 4.9: Distribution of gestational hypertension cases in patients who had single & recurrent abortions in the three age groups.

4.1.11 Abortion & diabetes mellitus

Six out of eighty seven aborted women suffered from gestational hyperglycemia, 5 (83.3 %) of them related to the recurrent abortion group and 1 (16.6 %) to the single abortion group, and those patients were develop abortion in the first and second trimester of the pregnancy. In the recurrent abortion group there were equal incidence (3.4%) of the development of diabetes mellitus in the ages between 26 to 35 and 36 to 45 years ($p > 0.05$),while when we compared them with the age group ≤15 to 25 we found that there was only 1 (1.7%) patients suffered from gestational hyperglycemia in this age group ,there is significant differences ($p < 0.05$) between this group and the other two age groups .For the single abortion group there was only 1 (3.4%) out of 29 patient develop diabetic mellitus during her pregnancy and related to the ages between 26 to 35 years. When we compared between single and recurrent abortion groups of the patients we found that there is highly significant differences (p <0.01) regarding the development of gestational hyperglycemia (Figure 4.10).

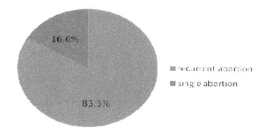

Figure 4.10: Distribution of diabetes mellitus cases in single and recurrent abortions.

4.1.12 Poly cystic ovarian syndrome (PCOs)

As we show in the figure (4.11), there were only 2 (3.4%) out of 58 patients with recurrent abortion suffered from polycystic ovarian syndrome which was diagnosed by gynecologist after they did to the patients the associated hormonal assay and ulterasonagraphy (abdominal and transveginal) .There is significant differences ($P < 0.05$) between single and recurrent abortion groups and significant differences ($P < 0.05$) between recurrent abortion and control groups.

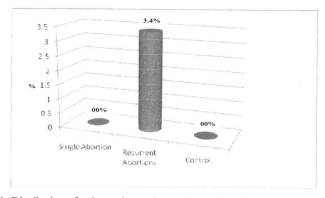

Figure 4.11: Distribution of poly cystic ovarian syndrome in patients with single or recurrent abortions and control groups.

4.1.13 Anomalies of the female genital tract

By doing abdominal ultrasonagraphy to the patients it had been found that there was 5(8.6%) out of 58 patients with recurrent abortions had abnormalities in their uterus, 2(40%) of them had bicornoated uterus, 1(20 %) had uterine fibroid &the other 2(40%) had septated uterus, while there is no such abnormalities was recorded in single abortion group. There is a significant differences (P <0.05) between recurrent and single abortion group (Figure 4.12).

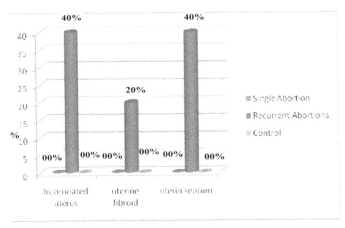

Figure 4.12: The distribution of the uterine anomalies (bicornoated uterus, uterine fibroid & septated uterus) in patients with single& recurrent abortions and control group.

4.1.14 Abortion and cervical incompetence

Cervical incompetence was positive in 6(6.8%) out of 87 cases of abortions, its higher incidence was recorded in recurrent abortions group (4.5%),while in single abortion group their incidence was (2.2%).There is significant differences(p< 0.05) between patients and control group and between recurrent and single abortion groups (p < 0.05)(Figure 4.13).

4.2 Laboratory investigations

4.2.1 Packed cell corpuscle

The mean & standard deviation of packed cell corpuscle (PCV) values in all aborted women (single & recurrent) & healthy control groups were within

Chapter Four ———————————————————————— Results

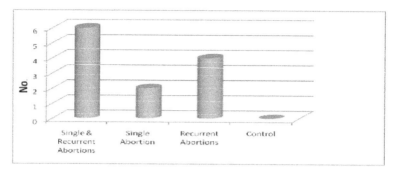

Figure 4.13: Cervical incompetence &its association with abortions in patients who had single, recurrent, single & recurrent abortions and control groups.

Table (4.2): Packed cell corpuscle (PCV) values in patients with abortions (single & recurrent) and control group.

Groups	Mean ± SD %
Single abortion	0.38 ± 0.01
Recurrent abortion	0.38 ± 0.02
Control	0.39 ± 0.02

normal ranges, and so there is no significant relationship (p >0.05) between anemia and abortion(Table 4.2).

4.2.2 Hemoglobin (Hb) concentrations

The table(4.3) represent the mean & standard deviation of hemoglobin values(Hb) in all aborted women & healthy control groups were within normal ranges, (p value >0.05).

Table (4.3): Mean & standard deviation of Hb value in patients with abortions (single & recurrent) and healthy control group.

Groups	Mean ± SD gm\dl
Single abortion	12.5 ± 0.6
Recurrent abortion	12.5 ± 0.7
Control	12.6 ± 0.7

4.2.3 Toxoplasmosis and its relation to abortions

From aborted women ,27 (31%) sera out of 87 were positive for antitoxoplasma antibodies, while 60 (68.9%) out of 87 sera of aborted women as well as control sera were negative for antitoxoplasma antibodies ,there were significant relationship ($p < 0.05$) between *Toxoplasma* infection and abortion(Figure 4.14).

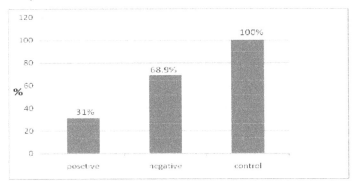

Figure (4.14): The distribution of the samples subjected to *Toxoplasma* infection.

4.2.3.1 The distribution of *Toxoplasma gondii* according to the number of patients

Out of 27 positive cases, 7 (25.9%) cases were with single abortion and 20 (74%) cases were with recurrent abortions, there is highly significant differences ($p < 0.01$) between single and recurrent abortions groups of the patients ,also there is significant differences($p < 0.05$) between abortions groups and control (Figure 4.15).

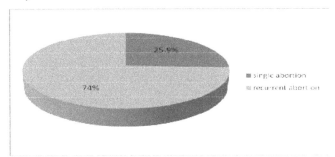

Figure (4.15): The distribution of the toxoplasma infection in patients with single and recurrent abortion.

4.2.3.2 The distribution of *Toxoplasma gondii* according to the age

Figure 4.16 illustrated the distribution of antitoxoplasma antibodies according to the age groups, which show that the highest number of the positive cases (18) was related to the age group ≤15 to 25 years, followed by (7) in the age group 26 to 35 years while the lowest number of these cases (2) was related to the age group 36 to 45 years. There is significant relationship ($p < 0.05$) between *Toxoplasma* infection and ages.

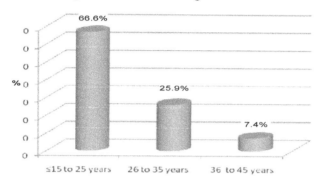

Figure (4.16): Distribution of *Toxoplasma gondii* infection according to the ages of the patients.

4.2.3.3 The distribution of *Toxoplasma* according to the trimesters of pregnancy

Figure 4.17 demonstrate the rate of infections according to the trimester of pregnancy, in single and recurrent abortion groups it was observed that the higher incidence of abortion was in the first trimester (62.9%), followed by second trimester abortion (37%), and the highest incidences of first trimester abortion was related to recurrent abortions group (44.4%), and also the highest incidence of second trimester abortion was related to the recurrent abortion group (29.6%) There were significant differences ($p < 0.05$) between single and recurrent abortions groups of the patients.

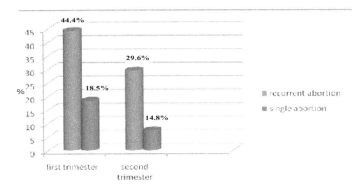

Figure (4.17): The distribution of the Toxoplasma infection in patients with single and recurrent abortion according to the time of abortion.

4.2.3.4 The distribution of *Toxoplasma gondii* according to the types of antibodies (IgM,IgG)

According to this study, the most common type of anti-*Toxoplasma* antibody in sero-positive cases was the IgM antibody which was found in 22 (81.4%) out of 27 sero-positive cases, while the IgG type was present in 5(18.5%)patients. There were significant differences ($p < 0.05$) between IgM and IgG types of antibodies. (Figure 4.18).

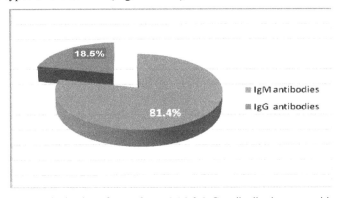

Figure (4.18): The distribution of *Toxoplasma* IgM & IgG antibodies in sero-positive cases.

4.2.4 Cytomegalovirus infection and it's relation to abortions

From aborted women ,15 (17.2%) sera out of 87 were positive for CMV antibodies, while 72 (82.7%) sera out of 87 aborted women as well as control sera were negative for CMV antibodies ,there were significant relationship ($p < 0.05$) between CMV infection and abortion(Figure 4.19).

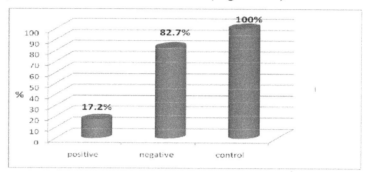

Figure (4.19): The distribution of the samples subjected to CMV infection.

4.2.4.1 The distribution of CMV infection according to the number of patients

We found in this study that the higher number of CMV infections was related to the patients with recurrent abortions which was 12(80%) out of 15 seroposetive cases,while in the single abortion the number of sero-positive cases was 3(20%) cases. There were significant differences ($p < 0.05$) between single and recurrent abortion groups of the patients (Figure 4.20).

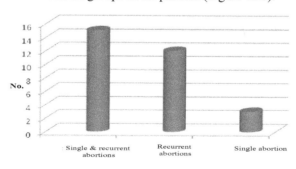

Figure (4.20): The distribution of CMV infection in patients with single, recurrent and single & recurrent abortions.

4.2.4.2 The distribution of CMV infections according to the ages

In this study we found that the higher incidence of CMV infections was related to the age group ≤15 to 25 years which was 9.1%, followed by the age group 26 to 35 years that had incidence of about 6.8%, while the age group 36 to 45 years had the lower incidence which was 1.1%. There were significant differences ($p < 0.05$) between these age groups (Figure 4.21).

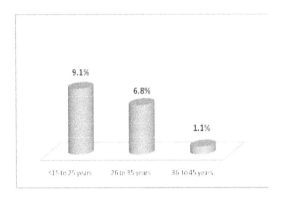

Figure (4.21): The distribution of CMV infection according to the ages of the patients.

4.2.4.3 The distribution of CMV infections according to the trimester of pregnancy

Out of 15 sero-positive cases, we found that CMV infections were responsible for 66.6% of first trimester abortion and 33.3% of second trimester abortion. There is significant differences ($p<0.05$) between first and second trimester abortion regarding CMV infections (Figure 4.22).

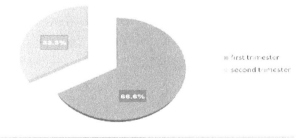

Figure (4.22): The distribution of the CMV infection according to the time of abortions (first and second trimester of abortions).

4.2.4.4 The distribution of CMV infections according to the types of antibodies (IgM, IgG)

According to this study, the most common type of anti CMV antibodies in sero-positive cases was the IgG antibody which was found in 9(60%) out of 15 sero-positive cases, while the IgM type was present in 6 (40%) of sero-positive cases (Figure 4.23).

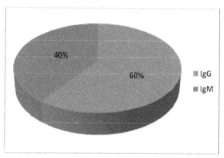

Figure (4.23): Distribution of anti-CMV (IgM & IgG) antibodies in sero-positive cases of abortion.

4.2.5 Rubella infection and its relation to abortions

There was no case had been recorded regarding anti-rubella IgM and IgG antibodies ($p > 0.05$) in both patients and control groups (Table 4.4).

4.2.6 Antiphospholipid antibodies and its relation with abortions

In this study there were 4 patients out of 87, had antiphosoholipid (IgM,IgG) antibodies in their sera ($p > 0.05$), 2 of them were related to single abortion group and 2 to the recurrent abortion group ($p > 0.05$), and all of them developed abortion in the first trimester of their pregnancy.

Regarding the type of antibodies, it was of IgM type and related to the patients who had single abortion and their ages run between ≤15 to 25 years. While in recurrent abortions group, one of the cases was related to the age between ≤15 to 25 years and had IgG type of antiphospholipid antibodies, and the other case had IgM type and related to the age between 26 to 35 years. There

Table 4.4: Frequency distribution of Rubella IgM & IgG antibodies in different ages related to the study groups

Groups			Age (years)					
			≤15-25		26-35		36-45	
			No.	%	No.	%	No.	%
Single abortion	First trimester	IgM	00	00%	00	00%	00	00%
		IgG	00	00%	00	00%	00	00%
	Second trimester	IgM	00	00%	00	00%	00	00%
		IgG	00	00%	00	00%	00	00%
Recurrent abortion	First trimester	IgM	00	00%	00	00%	00	00%
		IgG	00	00%	00	00%	00	00%
	Second trimester	IgM	00	00%	00	00%	00	00%
		IgG	00	00%	00	00%	00	00%
Control	First trimester	IgM	00	00%	00	00%	00	00%
		IgG	00	00%	00	00%	00	00%
	Second trimester	IgM	00	00%	00	00%	00	00%
		IgG	00	00%	00	00%	00	00%

is significant differences ($p < 0.05$) between abortions group and control group regarding the development of antiphosoholipid (IgM,IgG) antibodies (Table 4.5).

4.2 7 Anticardiolipin antibodies and its effect on abortions

Out of 87 cases of abortion, there were 3 cases positive for anticardiolipin IgM and IgG antibodies, and this result is significant when we compare it with control group ($p<0.05$). The higher incidence of the antibodies where in single abortion group (66.6%), which represented by two cases who developed first trimester abortion and both of them shown IgM types of antibody but one related to the age group ≤ 15 to 25 years and the other to the age group 26 to 35 years. Regarding recurrent abortions group there were only one (33 %) case shown IgG type of antibodies in their sera and she had also first trimester abortion and related to the age group 26 to 35 years. There is significant differences ($p<0.05$) between single and recurrent abortions group (Table 4.6).

Table 4.5: Frequency distribution of antiphospholipid (IgM & IgG) antibodies in different ages related to the study groups.

Groups			Age (years)					
			≤15-25		26-35		36-45	
			No.	%	No.	%	No.	%
Single abortion	First trimester	IgM	2	50%	00	00%	00	00%
		IgG	0	00%	00	00%	00	00%
	Second trimester	IgM	00	00%	00	00%	00	00%
		IgG	00	00%	00	00%	00	00%
Recurrent abortion	First trimester	IgM	00	00%	1	25%	00	00%
		IgG	1	25%	00	00%	00	00%
	Second trimester	IgM	00	00%	00	00%	00	00%
		IgG	00	00%	00	00%	00	00%
Control	First trimester	IgM	00	00%	00	00%	00	00%
		IgG	00	00%	00	00%	00	00%
	Second trimester	IgM	00	00%	00	00%	00	00%
		IgG	00	00%	00	00%	00	00%

Table 4.6: Frequency distribution of anticardiolipin IgM & IgG antibodies in different ages related to the study groups

Groups			<15-25 No.	<15-25 %	26-35 No.	26-35 %	36-45 No.	36-45 %
Single abortion	First trimester	IgM	1	33.3%	1	33,3%	00	00%
		IgG	00	00%	00	00%	00	00%
	Second trimester	IgM	00	00%	00	00%	00	00%
		IgG	00	00%	00	00%	00	00%
Recurrent abortion	First trimester	IgM	00	00%	00	00%	00	00%
		IgG	00	00%	1	33.3%	00	00%
	Second trimester	IgM	00	00%	00	00%	00	00%
		IgG	00	00%	00	00%	00	00%
Control	First trimester	IgM	00	00%	00	00%	00	00%
		IgG	00	00%	00	00%	00	00%
	Second trimester	IgM	00	00%	00	00%	00	00%
		IgG	00	00%	00	00%	00	00%

Chapter Five: Discussion

5.1 History of the patients

5.1.1 Age distribution in patients with abortion

According to this study we found that the higher incidence of single abortion (63.0%) was related to the ages between≤ 15 to 25 years while in the recurrent abortion groups we found that the higher incidence of abortion (53.4%) occurred in the age groups 26 to 35 years.

5.1.2 The distribution of patients with single & recurrent abortions according to age groups

The recurrent abortion group of the patients represents the higher percentage in all age group, and the most common cases of recurrent abortion (79.4%) were recorded in the ages between 26 to 35 years (Figure 4.2).

This is may be due to that with age the probability of occurrence of mutation of the chromosomes increase such as trisomy 21.

Or with age disturbance of hormones (Estradiol, Human chronic gonadotrophin (HCG) or progesterone hormone) may present which may lead to development of abortion.

Or with the progress of age the probability of exposure to environmental pollution increase and when these pollutants accumulate in the body it may have teratogenic effect on the developing embryo or fetus or the likelihood of occurrence of gestational hypertension increase with increase maternal age.

Also in this study we found the higher incidence of single abortion were 45.25% and related to the ages between ≤ 15 to 25 years.

This may be due to that in the ages between ≤ 15 to 25 years the female is in the highest level of activity and physical work, in contact with animal (especially the cat) as part of her job, that make her more liable for infection especially *Toxoplama* infection.

The result of this study is consist with many other studies(Abdella *et al.,* 1993; Munné *et al.* ,1995, ; Andersen *et al.,*2000 ;AL-Barwary, 2004*;* Heffner

,2004, AL-Jeboori, 2005)who observed that risk of spontaneous abortion increased with increasing maternal age.

Snijders *et al.* (1999) shown that the association of age of the mother and the increased likelihood of chromosomal abnormalities is manifested by the agerelated increase of trisomy 21.

Andersen *et al.* (2000) stated that at age 42 years, more than half of pregnancies resulted in fetal loss, the risk of a spontaneous abortion was 8.9% in women aged 20–24 years and 74.7% in those aged 45 years or more.

5.1.3 Age distribution in patients with single & recurrent abortions according to the time of abortion

We found in this study that higher incidence of the first trimester abortion was 71.42% and related to the age groups ≤ 15 to 25 years, there is significant differences ($p<0.05$) between the age group ≤ 15 to 25 and 36 to 45 years. For the second trimester abortion we found that it's incidence was nearly equal (50%) in the age groups 26 to 35 and 36 to 45 year (Figure 4.3).

This may be due to that in the ages between ≤ 15 to 25 years the female work in the house increase that make her more contact with the debris of the cats during her cleaning to the garden for example, and these feces or debris carry *Toxoplasma* parasite and this parasite cause first trimester abortion.

The finding of this study consists with that of Kadhim (2007) who found in his study that the higher incidence of abortion occurs in first trimester of pregnancy.

5.1.4 Family history of abortion

In this study we found that there is highly significant relationship between abortion and family history of abortion ($p < 0.01$), this may be due to that one of the causes of abortion is genetic.

These chromosomal abnormalities may transmit to the offspring, Jindal, (2007) demonstrated that chromosomal investigation of the couple may reveal abnormalities (only in 2-3 % of couple) in any of the parent.

5.1.5 Smoking prevalence in abortion

The smoking has adverse effect on pregnancy, as we found in this study, in which the incidence of smoking was 19.5% in single and recurrent abortion groups, and the highest one was in recurrent abortion group (20.6%) (Figure 4.7).

This can be explain by the fact that the chemical substance that present in smoke have many effects like, placental insufficiency, fetal hypoxia, increased carboxyhemoglobin levels, increased placenta-to-birth weight ratios, placenta previa, abruptio placentae, and reduced uterine and placental blood flow.

Another possible mechanism of the effects of smoking during pregnancy involves absorption of cyanide from cigarette smoke.

This results is in accordance with Mendola *et al.*, (1998) who did his study in Italy population and found that the risk of abortion is increased by 40% in smokers, while Neonatol (2000) found that the incidence of smoking during pregnancy in the US have ranged from 35-48%.

Also this study is in accordance with many other studies (Kline *et al.*, 1977; Windham *et al.*, 1992; Bulletin, 2001; Rasch, 2003).

While Kirsten *et al.* (2003) did not support findings from previous studies of an association between smoking and spontaneous abortion.

5.1.6 Rh-incompatability prevalence in abortion

There is significant relationship between abortion (single and recurrent) and Rh- incompatability as we found in this study, in which there were 4.9% of the patients incompatible with their husbands (Figure 4.8).

This may occur due to the presence of maternal embryotoxic anti-D antibodies in the blood of Rh- negative woman.

Rh refers to a group of protein molecules on the surface of the red blood cells that are unique to each person. Within this blood group, Rh0 (D) is the protein that usually causes incompatibility problems

Rh incompatibility refers to a difference between the Rh factor of a pregnant woman and that of her developing fetus, causing anti-Rh antibodies to develop and resulting in a serious, sometimes life-threatening reaction in the fetus (McLaughlin, 2006).

5.1.7 History of infertility

This study demonstrates that there is significant relationship between abortion (single and recurrent) and infertility (Table 4.1).

This may be due to that most of the pregnancy losses are unrecognized and occur before or during the next expected menses.

So the patient considered as infertile because her pregnancy unrecognized clinically.

This hypothesis has, in fact, been corroborated by the data collected by Wilcox *et al.*; (1988) they investigated the overall incidence of abortion by measuring daily urinary concentrations of human chorionic gonadotropin (hCG) during menstrual cycles.

With an hCG level above 0.025 ng/mL on 3 consecutive days as a criterion of early pregnancy, they found that 22% of pregnancies ended before pregnancy was clinically detected, and the clinically recognized loss rate was 12%. This finding is in accordance with the study that performed by Dhont (2003).

5.1.8 Abortion and hypertension

The relationship between hypertension and abortion is highly significant ($p < 0.01$) as we found in this study (Figure 4.9).

This may occur due to that elevated blood pressure can cause vasospasm, growth restriction, hypoxia, and abruptio placentae which adversely affect the developing embryo or fetus.

This finding is in accordance with many studies like Clifford *et al.,* 1994; Chong *et al.*, 1995; Marry and Stephenson, 1996).

5.1.9 Abortion & diabetes mellitus

It had been detected in this study that there was highly significant relationship (p<0.01) between recurrent abortion & diabetes mellitus (Figure 4.10), in which women with abortions (single &recurrent) had high fasting and postprandial glucose levels.

This may be due to that, poor control of preexisting or gestational diabetes during organogenesis (up to about 10 week's gestation) may lead to increase risk of major congenital malformations and then spontaneous abortion.

There are many studies that consist with this study like Dhont (2003), Montvale (2007) and Blackwell (2008)

But Mills *et al*. (1988) don't support this result; they enrolled 386 women with insulin-dependent diabetes and 432 women without diabetes before or within 21 days after conception and followed both groups prospectively. The incidence of pregnancy loss was the same in both groups (16.1% and 16.2%).

5.1.10 Poly cystic ovarian syndrome (PCOs)

The only two cases that were recorded in this study were related to the recurrent abortions group which had percentage of about 3.4% from all abortion cases (Figure 4.11).

This has been attributed to elevated levels of luteinising hormone (LH) that may produce an adverse environment for the oocyte, perhaps even inducing premature maturation and completion of the first meiotic division and also due to insulin resistance or excess androgens.

The results of this study consist with that of Jim *et al*. (2001) who suggested that the higher risk of spontaneous abortion observed in women with PCOS is likely to be due to their high prevalence of obesity and the type of treatment they receive.

5.1.11 Anomalies of the female genital tract

In this study the higher incidence of the female genital tract anomalies were recorded in the recurrent abortion group which was 8.6%, and there was a highly significant differences (p <0.01) between single and recurrent abortion groups (Figure 4.12).

This can be explained by the fact that in our society when the patient get abortion for the first time she do not try to do any investigation until she engaged onto the field of recurrent abortions stat.

This finding in accordance with many studies like Muckle *et al.*(2008) who found that the incidence of abortion due to uterine anomalies were vary from 0.13% to 4.0% ,also Christiansen *et al.*(2005) support this study where he found that uterine anomalies causes 15% of abortion. We conclude that the incidence of the female genital tract anomalies as cause of abortion in our city is double the incidence in other countries.

5.1.12 Abortion and cervical incompetence

In this study we found that cervical incompetence was responsible for 6.8% of abortion's incidence, single and recurrent, but the higher percentage (4.5%), was related to recurrent abortion group of the patients(Figure 4.13), there is significant differences (p <0.05) between single and recurrent abortion groups. This may be due to that cervical incompetence is one of the causes that required treatment, so if it not treated probably so recurrent abortion will result.

All of those patients develop abortion in the second trimester of their pregnancy. The explanation is that with the progression of the pregnancy, the pressure of the baby on the cervix will increase, and because of the weakness of the cervix, so abortion will take place. This result consists with many studies (Christiansen *et al.*, 2005; Reprod, 2006).

5.2 Laboratory investigations

5.2.1 Packed Cell Volume (PCV) count and Hemoglobin (Hb) concentrations

As we shown in the table (4.2) that all the values of PCV were in normal range, (p value >0.05) so we conclude that there is no association between anemia and abortion.

This is may be due to that most of the patients visit the hospital after about 6 month from her last abortion, so the storage of the body during this period returns to it's normal state.

5.2.2 Toxoplasmosis and it's relation to abortions

As we found in this study the Toxoplasma infection represent the cause number one of abortions, were the number of positive cases for antitoxoplasma antibodies were 27 (31%) cases (Figure 4.14), so the relationship between abortion and toxoplasma infection was highly significant ($p < 0.01$).

5.2.2.1 Distribution of *Toxoplasma gondii* according to number of patients

According to the results of this study we found that the highest number of positive cases for *Toxoplasma* antibody was related to recurrent abortions group which was 20(74%) cases, while the positive cases that related to single abortion was 7(25.%) cases(Figure 4.14).

This may be due to the fact that in our society when the woman develop abortion for the first time, she rarely visit the clinic looking for the cause of her abortion, so the parasite remain in latent state and again when the mother become pregnant where her immunity suppressed due to certain physiological changes in the body that occur during pregnancy so the parasite will reactivated again and become the cause of her next abortion in addition to the presence of another factors that act together with *T. gondii* parasite in killing the developing embryo or fetus.

This finding not in accordance with Christiansen *et al.*(2005), Mohammed (2008) who found that the higher incidence of positive cases were related to the single abortion group.

5.2.2.2 The distribution of Toxoplasma g*o*ndii according to the ages

This study shown that the highest number of positive cases for antitoxoplasma antibody was 18 and related to the ages between ≤15 to 25 years then the age groups 26 to 35 years and 36 to 45 years were their number of positive cases were 7 and 2 respectively (Figure 4.16).

This may explained by that the ages between ≤15 to 25 years represent the optimum period of fertility and reproduction and because the pregnancy reduce the immunity of the body thus this critical period of woman's life has higher chance for activation of latent infection of T.gondii that can be transmitted vertically to the fetus .

Also due to that in this ages the physical activity of the female increase such as cleaning the garden that make her in contact with the debris of the cats that contaminated with Toxoplasma oocytes .

The risk of transmition to the fetus is 15 % in the first trimester, 25 % in the second trimester and 65 % in the third trimester (Kapperud *et al.,* 1996; Dunn *et al.,* 1999) .The severity of fetal infection is greatest with first-trimester infection, and congenital defects are rarely seen if the infection occurs after 20 weeks of gestation (Hacker *et al.,* 2010).

According to the previous data we conclude that Toxoplasma infection is associated with age and this is verified statistically($p < 0.05$)and this result consistent with many other studies , as the study of Al-Doski (2000); Al-Ani (2004) and Mohammed (2008) in Iraq, Tabbara (1999) in Saudi Arabia and Coelho *et al.* (2003) in Brazil.

5.2.2.3 The distribution of Toxoplasma gondii according to the trimester of pregnancy

It is observed in this study that the higher incidence of abortion that occurred due to infection with Toxoplasma gondii developed in the first trimester of pregnancy which was 62.9% in both single and recurrent abortion groups of patients (Figure 4.17).

This result not consists with Mohammed (2008) who found that the higher incidence of abortion occurs in the second trimester of pregnancy. But consists with Hacker *et al.,* 2010.

5.2.2.4 The distribution of *Toxoplasma gondii* according to the type of antibodies

In this study it was recorded 27(31%) out of 87 cases of abortions who had antitoxoplasma IgM and IgG antibodies in their sera; but the most common antibodies was of IgM type and the number of cases that had IgM antibodies in their sera were 22(81.4%) cases,16 out of 22 case were related to recurrent abortions group and 6 were related to single abortion group (Figure 4.18).

Regarding IgG antibodies, the number of positive cases in this study were 5 (18.5%) out of 27 cases and also the highest number (5) were related to recurrent abortion group. There is significant differences ($p<0.05$) between single and recurrent abortion group regarding the type of antitoxoplasma antibodies in their sera.

5.2.3 Cytomegalovirus (CMV) infection and it's relation to abortion

The relationship between CMV infection and abortion as demonstrated by this study is significant ($p<0.05$) where the CMV infection represent the second most common causes of abortion in this study.

5.2.3.1 The distribution of CMV infection according to the number of patients

In this study we found that the higher number of CMV infections was related to the recurrent abortions group of the patients which was 12 cases out of 15 seroposetive cases (Figure 4.20).

This is can be explain by the fact that the cytomegalovirus is one of the viruses that remain latent in the body and reactivated again when the immunity of the body reduced during pregnancy, so there is vicious cycle that lead to recurrent abortion unless the treatment is received.

This result not in accordance with that of Mohammed (2008) who found that the number of positive cases for CMV antibodies were more in single abortion.

Chapter Five ——————————————————— Discussion

5.2.3.2 The distribution of CMV infection according to the ages

According to this study we found that CMV infection is more prevalence in patients whom ages range between ≤15 to 25 years where it's incidence was 53.3%, while the age group 26 to 35 years had an incidence of about 40% (Figure 4.21).

This may be due to that in the ages between ≤15 to 25 years the female in her optimum activity regarding her reproduction and fertility and because that she may had CMV infection which remained dormant in her body and because that during pregnancy the immunity of the body reduce so the latent cytomegalovirus will reactivated .This finding is in accordance with Schleiss, 2010 who found that two age groups have higher rates of acquisition of infection: toddlers who attend group daycare and adolescents.

5.2.3.3 The distribution of CMV infection according to the trimester of pregnancy

This study demonstrated that 66.6% of the CMV infections occur in the first trimester of pregnancy (Figure 4.22).This may be due to the fact that first trimester of the pregnancy is considered as a critical period in which the fetus is not well established in the uterus and it is threatened for abortion whenever the mother is expose to any risky factor such as reactivation of latent infection as CMV that result from immunosuppressant concomitant with pregnancy which can lead to placental infection and next placental insufficiency, with subsequent embryonic death.

Also CMV infection may induce genetically and anatomically abnormal embryo which is may considered as cause that leading to abortion in the first trimester of the pregnancy. This result consists with other many studies like Kadhim (2007) &Mohammed (2008).

5.2.3.4 The distribution of CMV infection according to type of antibodies

In this study we found that anti -CMV IgG antibodies had higher incidence, they presented in 10.3% of the sera of aborted women (Figure 4.23).

The presence of both anti-CMV (IgG &IgM) antibodies during pregnancy may be refer to reactivation of a previous latent infection as a result of immune suppression that occur during pregnancy or presence of other infection may also lead to reactivation of latent CMV infection.

This result was consisting with that of Kadhim (2007), who found that, 27.8% of the aborted women had anti -CMV IgG antibodies in their sera. While Abdulla, (2000) & Ali,(2001) found that IgM antibodies were more common than IgG antibodies in the sera of aborted women, and the incidences of these antibodies where 4.83% and 16.8% respectively.

5.2.4 Rubella infection and it's relation to abortion

In this study we detected that neither the patients group nor the control had anti rubella antibodies in their sera (Table 4.4).

But this result not consist with the study that performed by AL-Jeboori,(2005) where he found in his study that anti-rubella antibody where positive in 3.3% of the patients. This may be due to that in our society most of the females received the anti Rubella vaccine during their teenage, so those female develop immunity against rubella virus.

Other studies that not consist with this study are; Abdulla,(2000)and Turbadkar *et al.*,(2003).

5.2.5 Antiphospholipid antibodies and it's relation with abortion

In this study there were only 4 (4.5%) cases positive for antiphoshholipid IgM and IgG antibodies, all the patients had first trimester abortion(Table 4.5).

This may occur due to that these antiphospholipid antibodies react against proteins that bind to anionic phospholipids on plasma membranes of the trophoblast cells, which are involved in the establishment of uteroplacental vasculature and maintenance of placental blood fluidity .So thrombus will form result in defect in the implantation and subsequent placentation then abortion.

This result is in accordance with (Fabio *et al.*, 1991.; Rai *et al.*, 1995; Dhont, 2003; Mohammed, 2008).

From these data we conclude that the association between abortion (single and recurrent) and antiphospholipid antibodies is significant ($p < 0.05$).

5.2.6 Anticardiolipin antibodies and its effect on abortion

There were 3 (4.5%) cases positive for anticardiolipin antibodies, two cases developed first trimester abortion and both of them was show IgM types of antibody in their sera and related to single abortion group.

Regarding recurrent abortion group there were only one (33.3 %) case that was show IgG antibodies in their sera and she had also first trimester abortion (Table 4.6) .

There was no association between the presence of anticardiolipin antibody and spontaneous abortion.

This result is in accordance with the studies of Petri *et al*. (1987) and Couto& Barini, (1998), But Daboubi (2001) demonstrated an association between raised anticardiolipin antibodies and habitual abortion; he found in his study that high level of anticardiolipin antibodies activity was detected among 19.23% of the habitual abortion.

Conclusions and Recommendations

Conclusions

The higher incidence of single abortion (63.0%) was related to the ages between≤ 15 to 25 yea while in the recurrent abortion groups we found that the higher incidence of abortion (53.4%)occurred in the age groups 26 to 35 years.

2. The most common causes of abortion in this study was *Toxoplasma gondii* infection were the highest number of positive cases was related to recurrent abortion group and the higher incidence of abortion occurred in the first trimester of pregnancy.
3. Cytomegalovirus was the second most common cause of abortion, it was more prevalence in patients whom ages range between ≤15 to 25 years, and it was responsible for 66.6%of abortions that occurred in the first trimester of pregnancy.
4. Smoking has adverse effect on pregnancy, in which the incidence of smoking was 19.5% in single and recurrent abortion groups.
5. There was highly significant relationship ($p < 0.01$) between recurrent abortion & diabetes mellitus.
6. Cervical incompetence was responsible for 6.8% of abortion's incidence, single and recurrent.
7. All the patients with Antiphospholipid antibodies had first trimester abortion.

Conclusions and Recommendations

Recommendations

1. Measurement the level of HbA1c in the sera of aborted women which give us an idea about the level of glucose in the last two months.
2. Measurement the level of antithyriod antibody in the sera of aborted women, looking for any thyroid abnormality that associated with abortion.
3. As much as possible screening of most married girls before and during pregnancy for detection and treatment of *Toxoplasma*.
4. Health education of pregnant women about the mode of transmission and prevention of infection, by avoiding contact with cat feces, wearing disposable gloves during cleaning the garden, proper cooking of meat, washing of fruits, vegetables and proper hand washing.

References:

Abalovich, M.; Gutierrez, S.; Alcaraz, G.; Maccallini, G.; Garcia, A. and Levalle, O.(2002). Overt and subclinical hypothyroidism complicating pregnancy. 12(1):63-8.

Abdella, H.I. ; Burton, G. and Kirkland, A.(1993).: Age, pregnancy and miscarriage: uterine versus ovarian factors. Hum. Reprod. ;8:1512–1517.

Abdulla, S. F.(2000). Prevalence of Torch agents in complicated pregnancies. M.Sc . thesis, College of Medicine , University of Baghdad.

Abrão, R.A.; de Andrade, J.M. ;Tiezzi, D.G.; Marana, H.R.; Dos Reis, F.J. and Clagnan, W.S. (2007). "Treatment for low-risk gestational trophoblastic disease: Comparison of single-agent methotrexate, dactinomycin and combination regimens". Gynecologic Oncology 108 (1): 149.

Adler, S.P. (2007). Recent Advances in the Prevention and Treatment of Congenital Cytomegalovirus Infections. Seminars in Perinatology, 31(1): 10-18.

Al-Ani, S.K.(2004).Epidemiological and immunological study of toxoplasmosis among aborted women in Ramadi City. M.Sc. thesis. College of Medicine. Al-Anbar University.

Alaraji, S.M.H.(2010).Chromosomal Abnormalities Associated with Recurrent Spontaneous Abortions in Iraqi Women. BMJ,7:2-1.

AL–Barwary, M.K.N.(2004).Immunological and histopathological changes in women with spontaneous abortion. ph.D. Thesis, College of science, University of AL–Mustansiriya.

Al-Doski,B.D.A.(2000).Seroepidemiological study of toxoplasmosis among deferent groups of population in Duhok City by using Latex agglutination test and indirect hemoagglutination test .M.Sc. thesis, College of Medicine, Duhok University.

Aldrich, C.L.; Stephenson, M.D. and Karrison, T. (2001). HLA-G genotypes and pregnancy outcome in couples with unexplained recurrent miscarriage. Mol Hum Reprod, 12:1167–1172.

Alexander, D.; Wright, H. 0.; Nicholson ;Andrew, G. ; Taylor. And Betts,S. (1983). Spontaneous abortion and diabetes mellitus. Postgraduate Medical Journal ;59, 295-298.

AL-Hamadani , M . and Mahdi, N . (1997). Toxoplasmosis among women with habitual abortion . J . Eastern . Mediterranean. Health . 3 : 310-315 .

Ali , M . K . (2001) . Prevalence of human parvovirus B19 , Rubella , and CMV virus in complicated pregnancy. M.Sc. thesis, College of Medicine. University of Baghdad.

AL-Jeboori , M.J.H.(2005). Detection of some microorganisms accompanied to the recurrent abortions and its relationship with the blood group. M.Sc. Thesis, College of Science . AL-Mustansryia University.

Andersen, A.N; Wohlfahrt, J.; Christens, P. and Melbye, M. (2000). Maternal age and fetal loss: population based register linkage study, 320 (7251):1708.

Balasch , J .; Creus , M .; Fabregues , F .; Reverter , J .C. ; Carmona , F . and Tassies , J . (1996) . Antiphospholipid antibodies and human reproductive failure. Hum . Reprod . 11 : 2310-2315 .

Balasch, J.; Coll, O. and Martorell, J.(1996). Further data against HLA sharing in couples with recurrent spontaneous abortion. Gynecol Endocrinol. 1989;3:63 69.

Banatvala, J. E. and Brown, D.W.G. (2004). Rubella, The Lancet, 363(9415): 1127-1137.

Becker, G .J. and Hewiston, T.D. (2001). "Relaxin and renal fibrosis". Kidney Int. 59 (3): 1184–5.

Bellamy,K. ;Rousseau,S.A. and Gardner,S.P.(1986).The development of an M antibody capture ELISA for rubella IgM .J. Virol. Meth. ;14:243-251.

Best, J.M. (2007). "Rubella". Semin Fetal Neonatal Med 12 (3): 182–92.

Bhide, A. and Thilaganathan, B. (2004). "Recent advances in the management of placenta previa". Curr. Opin. Obstet. Gynecol.; 16 (6): 447–51.

Bianca,S. ; Barrano,B. ; Cutuli,N.; Indaco,L.; Ingegnosi,C.; Cataliotti, A.; Milana,G. and Ettore,G.(2010). "Recurrent pregnancy loss and inherited thrombophilia: who should be tested?" J. Clin. Pathol. ;61:1149-1150.

Blackwell, S. C. (2008). Diabetes Mellitus in Pregnancy (Gestational Diabetes), 4:44-46.

Bowie, W. R.; King, A. S.; Werker, D. H.; Isaac-Renton, J. L.; Bell, A. and Eng, S. B. (1997). Outbreak of Toxoplasmosis associated with municipal drinking water. Lanct. 350: 173-177.

Branch, D.W.; Porter, T.F and Paidas, M.J. (2001). Obstetric uses of Intravenous immunoglobulin: successes, failures, and promises allergy. Clin Immunol, 108: 133–138.

Bricker and Farquharson, R.G.(2002). Types of pregnancy loss in recurrent miscarriage: implications for research and clinical practice 17(5):1345-1350.

Bulletin. (2001). Management of recurrent early pregnancy loss. American. College of Obstetrics and Gynecology Practice 24:1–17.

Campbell, R.E.; Gaidamaka, G.; Han, S.K. and Herbison, A.E. (2009). "Dendro-dendritic bundling and shared synapses between gonadotropin-releasing hormone neurons". Proc. Natl. Acad. Sci. U.S.A. 106 (26): 10835–40.

Cardiol, A.C.(2009); Contraceptive Hormone Use and Cardiovascular Disease: Estrogen and Progesterone Physiology;53(3).

Carter, A.O. and Frank, J.W.(1986).congenital Toxoplasmosis; Epidemiological features and control., CAMJ., 135:618-623.

Caruso, C.; Buffa, S. and Candore, G. (2009). Mechanisms of immunosenescence ,6: 10.

Chan, P.D. and Johnson, S.M.(2006).Current clinical Strategies Gynecology and Obestetrics.

Chan-Ortega, J.(2007). Restore the Flow, 3(3):562.789.

Chen, Y.G.; Wang, Q.; Lin, S.L.; Chang, C.D.; Chuang, J.; Chung, J. and Ying, S.Y. (2006). "Activin signaling and its role in regulation of cell proliferation, apoptosis, and carcinogenesis". Exp. Biol. Med. (Maywood) 231 (5): 534–44.

Chong, P.; Matzner, W. and Ching, W. (1995). Immunology of recurrent spontaneous abortion. The female patient. 20: 1-5.

Christiansen, O.B.; Nybo Andersen, A.M. and Bosch, E. (2005). "Evidence-based investigations and treatments of recurrent pregnancy loss". Fertil. Steril.;83(4):821–39.

Clifford, K.; Rai, R.; Watson, H. and Regan, L. (1994). An informative protocol for the investigation of recurrent miscarriage : Preliminary experience of 500 consecutive cases. Hum. Reprod., 9 : 1328-1332.

Cnattingius, S.; Signorello, L.B. and Anneren, G. (2000). Caffeine intake and the risk of first-trimester spontaneous abortion. N Engl. J. Med., 343:1839–1845.

Coelho, R.A.; Kobayashi, M. and Carvalho, L.B. (2003). Prevalence of IgG antibodies specific to *Toxoplasma gondii* among blood donors in Recife. Notheast Brazil. Rev. Inst. Med. trop. S. Paulo., 45(4):229-231.

Cook, A.J.; Gilbert, R. F.; Buffolano, W.; Zuffereg, J.; Petersen, E. and Jenum, P. A. (2000). Source of *Toxoplasma* infection in pregnancy women : European multicentre case- control study. BMJ. 321 : 142-147.

Couto, E. and Barini, R. (1998). Anticardiolipin antibody in recurrent spontaneous aborting and fertile women, Sao Paulo Med. J. 116 (4): 1516-3180.

Daboubi, M.K.(2001). Anticardiolipin antibodies in women with recurrent abortion ,7(12):95-99.

Daniel,w.w.(1999).Propability and t-disterbution. Biostatistic.A Foundation for analysis in the health sience.7th editions;83-123.

Delhanty, J.D.; Harper, J.C. and Ao, A.(1997). Multicolour FISH detects frequent chromosomal mosaicism and chaotic division in Genet.; 99:755–760.

Dewick, P. M. (2002). Medicinal natural products: a biosynthetic approach. New York: Wiley. pp. 244.

Dhont M. (2003). Current Women's Health Reports, 3:361–366.

Diejomaoh, M. F.; AL –Azemi, M. M.; Bandar, A.; Egbase, PE. and Jirous, J. (2002). A favorable outcome of pregnancies in women with primary and recurrent pregnancy loss associated with antiphospholipid syndrome . Obstet . Gyncol . 266 : 61-66

Dimitrova, V.; Markov, D.and Dimitrov, R. (2007). "[3D and 4D ultrasonography in obstetrics]" (in Bulgarian). Akush Ginekol (Sofiia) 46 (2): 31–40.

DiPiro.(2007). Pharmacotherapy: A Pathophysiologic Approach. Chapter 82, page 1313.

Duff, P. A. (2007).Thoughtful Algorithm for the Accurate Diagnosis of Primary CMV Infection in Pregnancy. American Journal of Obstetrics and Gynecology, 196: 196-197.

Dungan, H.M.;Clifton, D.K.and Steiner, R.A. (2006). "Minireview: kisspeptin neurons as central processors in the regulation of gonadotropin-releasing hormone secretion". Endocrinology 147 (3): 1154–8.

Dunn , D .; Wallon , M .; Peyron , F .; Petersen , E . Pechham , C . and Gilbert , R . (1999) . Mother – to child transmission of toxoplasmosis : Risk estimates for clinical counselling . Lanct . 353 : 1829-1833 .

Everett, C. (1997). "Incidence and outcome of bleeding before the 20th week of pregnancy: prospective study from general practice.". BMJ 315 (7099): 32–4.

Fabio,P. ; Barbara,A.; David,F.; Massimo,L.; Guido, M. and Sergio,C.(1991). Antiphospholipid Antibodies and Recurrent Abortion ,77 (6):5.

Finer, L. B. and Henshaw,SK.(2003). Abortion Incidence and Services in the United States in 2000. Perspectives on Sexual and Reproductive Health, 35:6–15.

Fowler, P.A. ; Sorsa-Leslie, T.; Harris, W. and Mason, H.D. (2003). "Ovarian gonadotrophin surge-attenuating factor (GnSAF): where are we after 20 years of research?" Reproduction, 126: 689–699.

Franceschini, I.; Lomet, D.; Cateau, M.;Delsol, G.; Tillet, Y.and Caraty, A.(2006). "Kisspeptin immunoreactive cells of the ovine preoptic area and arcuate nucleus co-express estrogen receptor alpha". Neurosci. Lett. 401 (3): 225–30.

Francois, K.E.and Foley, M.R. (2007). Antepartum and postpartum hemorrhage. In: Gabbe SG, Niebyl JR, Simpson JL, eds. Obstetrics - Normal and Problem Pregnancies. 5th ed. Philadelphia, Pa: Elsevier Churchill Livingstone;:chap 18.

Gibson, C.L.; Gray, L.J.; Bath, P.M. and Murphy, S.P. (2008). "Progesterone for the treatment of experimental brain injury; a systematic review". Brain 131 (2): 318–28.

Gonzalez-Gonzalez, N.L. ; Ramirez, O. and Mozas, J.(2008). Factors influencing pregnancy outcome in women with type 2 versus type 1 diabetes mellitus. Acta. Obstet. Gynecol. Scand ; 87:43.

Goodson, III. W.H.; Handagama, P.; Moore, II. D.H. and Dairkee, S. (2007). "Milk products are a source of dietary progesterone". 30th Annual San Antonio Breast Cancer Symposium. pp. 2028.

Graaff,V.D. (2006). Human Anatomy. Sixth Edition.

Gracia, C.; Sammel, M. ;Chittams, J.; Hummel, A.; Shaunik , A. and Barnhar, K. (2005). "Risk factors for spontaneous abortion in early symptomatic first-trimester pregnancies". Obstet Gynecol 106 (5 Pt 1): 993–9.

Grangeot-Keros, L.(1992).Rubella and pregnancy Path.Biol.;40:706-710.

Greenberg, J.S.; Clint, E. B. and Sarah, C. C. (2007). Exploring the dimensions of human sexuality (3rd ed.). 136–137.

Grossman, C.M. ; Morton, W.E. and Nussbaum, R.H.(1996). Hypothyroidism and spontaneous abortions among Hanford, Washington, downwinders. 51(3):175-6.

Guerina , N . G .; Hsu , H . W .; Meissner , H . C .; Maguire , J. H.; Lynfield , R . and Stechenberg , B . (1994) . Neonatal serologic screening and early treatment for congenital *Toxoplasma gondii* infection . N . Engl . J . Med . 330 : 1858-1863 .

Guyton,A.C. and Hall, J.E.(2006).Text book Of Medicale Physiology.11th edition.W.B.Saunders company,Philadilphia;1011-1026.

Hacker,N.F.; Gambone, J.C. and Hobel, C.J.(2010). Essential of obstetrics and Gynicology.5th edition. W.B. Saunders company ;208-213.

Hannafin,B. ; Lovecchio,F. and Blackburn, P.(2006).Do Rh-negative women with first trimester spontaneous abortion need Rh immunoglobulin? ,American Journal of Emergency Medicine.487-89.

Heffner, L. (2004).Advanced Maternal Age – How old is too old? New England Journal of Medicine; 351(19):1927–29.

Hines, T. (2001). "The G-Spot: A modern gynecologic myth". Am. J. Obstet. Gynecol. 185 (2): 359–62.

Homburg, R. (2008). The Mechanism of OvulationGlob. libr. women's med., 1756-2228.

Hu, L. ; Gustofson, R.L. and Feng, H. (2008). "Converse regulatory functions of estrogen receptor-alpha and -beta subtypes expressed in hypothalamic gonadotropin-releasing hormone neurons". Mol. Endocrinol. 22 (10): 2250–9.

Hughes, E.; Collins, J. and Vandekerckhove, P. (2007). Gonadotropin releasing hormone analogue as an adjunct to gonadotropin therapy for clomiphene-resistant polycystic ovariansyndrome. Cochrane Database Syst. Rev. ; 2: 97.

Hughes,G. (2009). Understanding Hughes Syndrome: Case Studies for Patients. Springer, 33:112-115.

Iams, J.D.; Romero, R.; Culhane, J.F. and Goldenberg, R.L. (2008). "Primary, secondary, and tertiary interventions to reduce the morbidity and mortality of preterm birth". Lancet 371 (9607): 164–75

Isachenko, V.; Lapidus, I .and Isachenko, E. (2009). "Human ovarian tissue vitrification versus conventional freezing: morphological, endocrinological, and molecular biological evaluation.". Reproduction 138: 319–27.

Jannini, E.; Simonelli, C. and Lenzi, A. (2002). "Sexological approach to ejaculatory dysfunction.". Int. J .Androl. 25 (6): 317–23.

Jim, X. ; Wang,1. ; Davies, M. J. ; and Norman ,R.J.(2001). Polycystic ovarian syndrome and the risk of spontaneous abortion following assisted reproductive technology treatment. 16(12): 2606-2609.

Jindal, U.N.(2007)." Recurrent Pregnancy Loss ",7235:5.

Kadhim,R.(2007). The role of some immunological changes and some viral infection in single and recurrent spontaneous abortion. ph.D thesis, College of science, University of Baghdad.

Kapperud , G .; Jenum , P . A.; Stray-Pedersen, B .; Melby , K . K .and Eskild, A . (1996). Risk factors for *Toxoplasma gondii* infection in pregnancy , results of a prospective case- control study in Norway. Am . J. Epidemiol. 144 : 405- 412 .

Karcaaltincaba, D. ; Sencan, I.; Kandemir,O. ; Guvendag-Guven,E. and Yalvac, S.(2010). Does brucellosis in human pregnancy increase abortion risk? Presentation of two cases and review of literature. Journal of Obstetrics and Gynecology Research, 36(2): 418–423.

Kaufman, M. H.; Stead,L. and Robert,F. (2007). First aid for the obstetrics & gynecology clerkship. New York: McGraw-Hill, Medical Pub. Division. pp. 138

Kearns, A.M.; Turner, A.J.; Eltringham, G.J. and Freeman, R. (2002). "Rapid detection and quantification of CMV DNA in urine using LightCycler-based real-time PCR". J. Clin. Virol. 24 (1-2): 131–4

Khan, G.Q. and Heggen, D. (1998). Recurrent Miscarriage ;OBGYN.net: The Universe of Women's Health

Khandekar, R. ;Sudhan ,A. ; Jain, B.K.; Shrivastav, K. and Sachan ,R. (2007). "Pediatric cataract and surgery outcomes in Central India: a hospital based study". Indian J. Med. Sci. 61 (1): 15–22.

Khattab, S.; Mohsen, I.A. ; Foutouh, I.A.; Ramadan ,A.; Moaz ,M. ; Al-Inany, H. (2006). Metformin reduces abortion in pregnant women with polycystic ovary syndrome. 22(12):680-4.

Kimball, J.W.(2010).Kimball's Biology Pages .http://biology-pages.info.

Kirsten,W.; Ulrik,K.; Brink,H.T.; Morten,H. and Jørgen S.N. (2003).A prospective study of maternal smoking and spontaneous abortion; 82(10):, 936-941

Kline, J., Stein, Z.A.; Susser, M. and Warburton, D. (1977) ". Smoking: A Risk Factor for Spontaneous Abortion "N. Engl. J. Med. 297:793–796.

Kutteh, W.H.(2006).Antiphospholipid antibody-associated recurrent pregnancy loss: treatment with heparin and low-dose aspirinis superior to low-dose aspirin alone. Obstet Gynecol,10:3301–3304

Lan, C.;Xiao, W.;Xiao-Hui, D.; Chun-Yan, H. and Hong-Ling, Y. (2008). "Tissue culture before transplantation of frozen-thawed human fetal ovarian tissue into immunodeficient mice". Fertil. Steril. PMID 19108826

Lanasa, M.C.; Hogge, W.A. and Kubik, C.J.(2001).A novel X chromosome-linked genetic cause of recurrent spontaneous abortion. Am. J. Obstet. Gynecol., 185:563–568.

Lawrence, J.M. ; Contreras, R. ; Chen, W. and Sacks, D.A.(2005). Trends in the prevalence of preexisting diabetes and gestational diabetes mellitus among a racially/ethnically diverse population of pregnant women. Diabetes Care 2008; 31:899.

Lee, Y.L. ; Ng, H. P. ; Laub, K. S. ; Liu, W. M. ; Wai Sum ,W. ; Yeung, W. S. B. and Kung, A.W.C.(2009). Increased fetal abortion rate in autoimmune thyroid disease is related to circulating TPO autoantibodies in an autoimmune thyroiditis animal model. 91(5): 2104-2109.

Leviton, A. and Cowan , L .(2002). A review of the literature relating caffeine consumption by women to their risk of reproductive hazards. Food Chem. Toxicol , 40:1271–1310.

Lewis,S.M.;Bain,B.J.and Bates,I.(2006). Dacie and Lewis Practical heamatology. 10[th]edition. Churchill Living stone Elsevier. Germany

Lim , K . J . H.; Odukoya , O . A .; Li , T. C . and Cooke , I .D. (1996) . Cytokines and immuno- endocine factors in recurrent miscarrige . Hum . Reprod. Update. 2 : 469-481 .

Losos, J. B.; Raven, P. H.; Johnson, G. B. and Singer, S. R. (2002). Biology. New York: McGraw-Hill. 1207–09.

Malm,G. and Engman,M.(2007). Congenital cytomegalovirus infections. Seminars in Fetal and Neonatal Medicine, 12(3): 154-159.

Marry, D. and Stephenson, M. (1996). Frequency of factors associated with habitual abortion in 197 couples. Fertil. Steril. 66: 24-28.

Mastenbroek, S. ;Twisk ,M.; van Echten-Arends, J.; Sikkema-Raddatz ,B. ; Korevaar, J.C. and Verhoeve, H.R. (2007). In vitro fertilization with preimplantation genetic screening. N. Engl. J. Med. ;357(1):9-17.

McGregor, D.G. (2000).Occupational exposure to trace concentrations of waste anesthetic gases. Mayo. Clin. Proc. ;75(3):273-7.

McLaughlin, E.(2008). Rh incompatibility, Marshall Medical Centers.

Mechoulam ,R. ; Brueggemeier, R.W. and Denlinger, D.L. (2005). Estrogens in insects. Cellular and Molecular Life Sciences 40 (9): 942-944.

Mendola ,P. ; Moysich, K.B; Freudenheim, J.L. ; Shields, P.G. ;Schisterman, E.F. ;Graham, S. ; Vena, J.E. ; Marshall, J.R. and Ambrosone, C.B.(1998). Risk of recurrent spontaneous abortion, cigarette smoking, and genetic polymorphisms in NAT2 and GSTM1, 9(6): 66-668.

Mills, J.L; Simpson ,J.L and Driscoll , S.G(1988) Incidence of spontaneous abortion among normal women and insulin-dependent diabetic women whose pregnancies were identified within 21days of conception. N Engl. J. Med., 319:1617–1623.

Moffett, A.; Regan, L. and Braude, P. (2004). "Natural killer cells, miscarriage, and infertility". BMJ.; 329(7477):1283–5.

Mohammed, G.J.(2008)."A study the role Toxoplasmosis ,cytomegalovirus and anti-phospholipids antibodies in cases abortion among women in Hilla city". M.Sc. thesis. College of Medicine. Babylon University

Monga,A.(2006).Gynaecology by Ten Teachers.18th edition.92-102.

Montvale, N.J. (2007)."Miscarriage: Causes of Miscarriage"... The PDR Family Guide to Women's Health and Prescription Drugs.: Medical Economics. pp. 345–50.

Mookerjee, I.; Solly, N.; Royce, S.; Tregear, G.;Samuel, C. and Tang, M. (2006). "Endogenous relaxin regulates collagen deposition in an animal model of allergic airway disease". Endocrinology 147 (2): 754–61.

Muckle, C.; Feinberg, E. and Glob, L. (2008). Developmental Abnormalities of the Female Reproductive Organs, women's med., 10 (3843): 1756-2228.

Munné, S.; Alikani, M. and Tomkin, G.(1995). Embryo morphology, developmental rates and maternal age are correlated with chromosome abnormalities. Fertil. Steril., 64:382–391.

Nardo, L.G.; Rai, R. and Backos, M.(2002). High serum luteinizing hormone and testosterone concentrations do not predict pregnancy outcome in women with recurrent miscarriage .Fertil. Steril., 77:348–352.

Navarrete-Palacios, E.; Hudson, R. and Reyes-Guerrero, G. (2003). "Lower olfactory threshold during the ovulatory phase of the menstrual cycle." Biological Psychology 63 (3): 269–279.

Neonatol, S. (2000). Review Perinatal complications associated with maternal tobacco use. 5(3):231-41.

Nielsen, M.;Barton, S.;Hatasaka, H. and Stanford, J. (2001). "Comparison of several one-step home urinary luteinizing hormone detection test kits to OvuQuick". Fertil. Steril.; 76(2):384–7.

Norwitz, M.D. and Errol, R. (2007). "Patient information: Postterm pregnancy".http://patients.uptodate.com/topic.asp?file=pregnan/5708.

Pan, D.S.; Liu, W.G.; Yang, X.F. and Cao, F. (2007). "Inhibitory effect of progesterone on inflammatory factors after experimental traumatic brain injury". Biomed. Environ. Sci. 20 (5): 432–8.

Pattision , N . S .; Chamley , L . W .; Liggins , G . C .; Buller , W . S. and Mckay , E . J . (1998) . Antiphospholipid antibodies in pregnancy : Prevalence and clinical . Br . J . Obstet . Gynecol . 100: 909-913 .

Patton , P . E . (1994) . Anatomic uterine defects . Clin Obstet Gynecol , 37 : 705-721.

Persson, M. ;Norman, M.and Hanson, U.(2009). Obstetric and perinatal outcomes in type 1 diabetic pregnancies: A large, population-based study. Diabetes Care; 32:2005.

Petri, M. ; Mitchell Golbus,M.; Robert Anderson, R.; Whiting-O'Keefe,Q.; Corash,L. and Hellmann, D.(1987). Antinuclear antibody, lupus anticoagulant, and anticardiolipin antibody in women with idiopathic habitual abortion. A controlled, prospective study of forty-four women. 21205.

Pfeiffer, K.A.; Fimmers, R. and Engels, G. (2001). The HLA-G genotype is potentially associated with idiopathic recurrent spontaneous abortion. Mol. Hum. Reprod, 7:373–378.

Potts , M .; Diggory , P . and Pell , J . (1997). Abortion . Great . Britain .

Pratt, D.; Novonty, M. and Kaberlein, G. (1993). Antithyroid antibodies and the association with nonorgan specific antibodies in recurrent pregnancy loss. Am. J. Obstet. Gynecol,168:837 -841.

Prechtl and Heinz .(2007). "Prenatal and Early Postnatal Development of Human Motor Behavior" in Handbook of brain and behavior in human development, Kalverboer and Gramsbergen eds., 415–418

Prossnitz ,E.R.; Arterburn, J.B. and Sklar, L.A. (2007). "GPR30: A G protein-coupled receptor for estrogen". Mol. Cell. Endocrinol, 138(42):265-266.

Qasim, S.M. ;Callan, C. and Choe, J.K. (1996). "The predictive value of an initial serum beta human chorionic gonadotropin level for pregnancy outcome following in vitro fertilization." Journal of Assisted Reproduction and Genetics 13 (9): 705–8.

Rai, R.; Backos, M.; Rushworth, F. and Regan, L. (2000).Polycystic ovaries and recurrent miscarriage: a reappraisal. Hum. Reprod.,15:612–615.

Rai, R.S. (1995). High prospective fetal loss rate in untreated pregnancies of women with recurrent miscarriage and antiphospholipid antibodies. Human reproduction, 10:3301–4.

Rana, A. ; Pradhan,N.; Gurung, G. and Singh, M. (2004).Induced septic abortion: A major factor in maternal mortality and morbidity Journal of Obstetrics and Gynaecology Research.

Rao,R.C. ; Lakshmi,A. and Sadhnani,M.D. (2008). Prevalence of hypothyroidism in recurrent pregnancy loss in first trimester,62(9):357-361.

Rasch, V. (2003). Cigarette, alcohol, and caffeine consumption: risk factors for spontaneous abortion. Acta Obstet. Gynecol. Scand, 82:182–188.

Rauch ,J. (1999) . Clinical detection of antiphospholipid antibodies In : Janof Liposome . New . York . P : 181-203 .

Regan, L.; Braude, P.R. and Trembath, P.L.(1989).Influence of postreproductive performance on risk of spontaneous abortion. Br Med J, 299:541–545.

Repord ,S. (2006). Anatomic Factors in Recurrent Pregnancy Loss:

Robert, F.P.; Karen, B.F.; Suresh, B.B.; William, J.B. and Stagno,S.(2006). Seminars in Fetal and Neonatal Medicine,12(3):154-159.

Roberts, S.; Havlicek, J.; Flegr, J.; Hruskova, M.; Little ,A.; Jones, B.;Perrett, D. and Petrie, M. (2004). "Female facial attractiveness increases during the fertile phase of the menstrual cycle". Proc .Biol. Sci. 7 (271 Suppl 5:S): 270–2.

Rodger, M.A. (2008).Inherited Thrombophilia and Pregnancy Complications. Revisited. Obstet Gynecol, 112:320-324.

Roof,R.L. and Hall, E.D. (2000). "Gender differences in acute CNS trauma and stroke: neuroprotective effects of estrogen and progesterone". J. Neurotrauma 17 (5): 367–88.

Ryan, K.J. and Ray, C.G . (2004). Sherris Medical Microbiology (4th ed.). McGraw Hill. pp. 556; 566–9.

Ryan, K.J. (1982). Biochemistry of aromatase: significance to female reproductive physiology. Cancer Res. 42 (8 Suppl): 3342s–3344s.

Sant-Cassia, L.J.(1985). Recurrent Abortion. Progress in Obstetrics and Gynecology. Edinburgh: Churchill-Livingstone; 5:248 258.

Scanlon,V.C. and Sanders,T.(2006). Essentials of Anatomy and Physiology. Fourth Edition

Schenker, J.G. and Margalloth, E.J. (1982). Intrauterine adhesions: an updated appraisal. Fertil. Steril.,37:593- 610.

Schindler, A.E.; Campagnoli, C.; Druckmann, R.; Huber, J.; Pasqualini, J.R.; Schweppe, K.W. and Thijssen, J.H. (2003). "Classification and pharmacology of progestins". Maturitas 46 Suppl 1: S7–S16.

Schleiss, M.R .(2010). "Acquisition of human cytomegalovirus infection in infants via breast milk: natural immunization or cause for concern?". Rev. Med. Virol. 16 (2): 73–82.

Scott, J.R. (1989). Habitual abortion: Recommendations for a reasonable approach to an enigmatic problem. 95:106.

Sharp, M. and Crop D.(2009). Spontaneous Abortion(Miscarriage).a subsidiary of Merck & Co., Inc., White house Station, N.J.

Shaw, J.L.; Dey, S.K.; Critchley, H.O. and Horne, A.W. (2010). "Current knowledge of the aetiology of human tubal ectopic pregnancy". Hum Reprod Update 16 (4): 432–44.

Siegel, M.; Fuerst, H.T. and Guinee, V.F .(1971). "Rubella epidemicity and embryopathy. Results of a long-term prospective study". Am. J. Dis. Child. 121 (6): 469–73.

Simpson, J.L.; Carson, S.A. and Mills, J.L.(1996).Prospective study showing that antisperm antibodies are not associated with pregnancy losses. Fertil. Steril., 66:36–42.

Simpson, J.L. and Bombard, A. (1987). Chromosomal abnormalities in spontaneous abortion, pathology, and genetic counselling. In Benner, M.J. & Edmond, D.K. (eds). Spontaneous and recurrent abortion .Oxford, Blackwell Scientific Publications: 51-76.

Singh, S . (2003) . Mother- to child transmission and diagnosis of *Toxoplasma gondii* infection during pregnancy . Ind . J . Med. Microbiol . 21 : 69-76 .

Slama, R. ; Bouyer, J. ; Windham, G. ; Fenster, L. ; Werwatz, A. and Swan, S. (2005). "Influence of paternal age on the risk of spontaneous abortion.". Am. J. Epidemiol ;161 (9): 816–23.

Snijders, R.J.; Sundberg ,K.and Holzgreve, W.(1999).Maternal age and gestation-specific risk for trisomy 21: effect of previous affected pregnancy. Ultrasound Obstet. Gynecol., 13:167–170.

Spence, D. and Melville, C. (2007). "Vaginal discharge". BMJ 335 (7630): 1147–51.

Staras ,S.A.; Dollard ,S.C.; Radford, K.W.; Flanders, W.D.; Pass, R.F. and Cannon ,M.J .(2006). "Seroprevalence of cytomegalovirus infection in the United States, 1988-1994". Clin. Infect. Dis. 43 (9): 1143–51.

Stegmann ,B.J. and Carey, J.C. (2002). "TORCH Infections. Toxoplasmosis, Other (syphilis, varicella-zoster, parvovirus B19), Rubella, Cytomegalovirus (CMV), and Herpes infections". Curr Women's Health Rep. ,2 (4): 253–8.

Stein -Carter,J.(2004). Reproductive Physiology, Conception, Prenatal Development.carterjs@uc.edu.

Stenchever ,M.A; Droegemueller, W; Herbst, A.L. and Mishell, D.R. (2001) Spontaneous and recurrent abortion. In: Comprehensive Gynecology, edn 4:280–299.

Stephenson, M.D.; Awartani, K.A. and Robinson, W.P. (2002). Cytogenetic analysis of miscarriages from couples with recurrent miscarriage: a case controlled study. Hum. Reprod.;17:446–451.

Stirrat, G.M. (1990). Recurrent miscarriage; definition and epidemiology. Lancet, 348, 1402–1406.

Stovall and Thomas, G. (2004). "Postdate Pregnancy". Durham Obstetrics and Gynecology. erythematosus. Journal of obstetrics and gynaecology, 5:207–9.

Stray-Pedersen, B.and Stray-Pedersen, S.(1984). Etiologic factors and abortion. Am. J. Obstet. Gynecol., 185:563–568.

Su, L.L. (2005). A prospective, randomized comparison of vaginal misoprostol versus intra-amniotic prostaglandins for mid-trimester termination of pregnancy. Am J Obstet Gynecol. ;193(4):1410-4.

Sulyok, S. ; Wankell, M. ; Alzheimer, C. and Werner, S. (2004). "Activin: an important regulator of wound repair, fibrosis, and neuroprotection". Mol. Cell. Endocrinol. 225 (1-2): 127–32.

Susan ,B.; Sarah, A.and Kathleen, S. (2004). "Women's sexual experience during the menstrual cycle: identification of the sexual phase by noninvasive measurement of luteinizing hormone". Journal of Sex Research ;41 (1): 82–93.

Tabbara, K.F. ; Al-Omar, O.M. ; Tawfic,A. and AL-Shammary, F. (1999).Toxoplasmosis in Saudi Arabia. Saudi Med.J., 20(1):46.

Temple, R.; Aldridge, V. and Greenwood, R.(2002). Association between outcome of pregnancy and glycaemic control in early pregnancy in type 1 diabetes: population based study. BMJ; 325:1275.

Thomas ,M.(1999). Cytogenetic basis of Recurrent abortions , Perinatology, 1 (4) : 181-187.

Tracy,S.(2005)." Having a Great Birth in Australia ed. David Vernon", Australian College of Midwives, 22.

Turbadkar , D .; Mathur , M . and Rele ,M. (2003) . Sero- prevalence of Torch infection in bad obstetric history . Ind. J . Med . Microbiol 21: 108-110.

Usui, R. ; Matsubara, S. and Ohkuchi, A. (2007). "Fetal heart rate pattern reflecting the severity of placental abruption". Archives of Gynecology and Obstetrics ;277 (3): 249.

van Zonneveld, P. ; Scheffer, G.; Broekmans, F. ; Blankenstein ,M. ; de Jong, F. ; Looman ,C. ;Habbema, J. and te Velde, E. (2003). "Do cycle disturbances explain the age-related decline of female fertility? Cycle characteristics of women aged over 40 years compared with a reference population of young women". Hum Reprod 18 (3): 495–501.

Voller,A. ;Bidwell ,D. ;Bartlett ,A. ;Flick ,D. ;Perkins ,M. and Oladshin, B. (1976).A Microplate Enzyme-immunoassay for *Toxoplasma* antibodies. J. Clin. Path.29:150-153.

Walter, F.(2003). Medical Physiology: A Cellular And Molecular Approaoch. Elsevier/Saunders. pp. 1300.

Wang, J.X.; Davies, M.J. and Norman, R.J.(2002). Obesity increases the risk of spontaneous abortion during infertility treatment. Obes. Res., 10:551–554.

Wang, X. ;Chen, C.; Wang, L. ;Chen, D. ;Guang ,W. and French, J. (2003). "Conception, early pregnancy loss, and time to clinical pregnancy: a population-based prospective study.". Fertil. Steril.; 79 (3): 577–84.

Weisinger, H.S. and Pesudovs, K. (2002). "Optical complications in congenital rubella syndrome". Optometry 73 (7): 418–24.

Weng, X.; Odouli, R.andLi, D.K.(2008).Maternal caffeine consumption during pregnancy and the risk of miscarriage: a prospective cohort study. Am. J. Obstet. Gynecol. ;198(3):279.e1-8.

Weschler, T.(2002). Taking Charge of Your Fertility (Revised ed.). New York: HarperCollins. 359–361.

Wilcox, A.J.; Baird, D.D. and Weinberg, C.R. (1999). "Time of implantation of the conceptus and loss of pregnancy.". New England Journal of Medicine 340 (23): 1796–1799.

Wilcox, A.J; Weinberg, C.R and Conner, J.F. (1988) .Incidence of early loss of pregnancy. N Engl J Med, 319:189–194.

Wilkinson, T.N.; Speed, T.P.; Tregear, G.W. and Bathgate, R.A .(2005). "Evolution of the relaxin-like peptide family". BMC evolutionary biology 5 (1): 14.

Windham, G.C.; Swan, S.H. and Fenster, L. (1992). "Parental Cigarette Smoking and the Risk of Spontaneous Abortion ".Am. J. Epidemiol, 135: 1394–1403.

WÖhrle,R. ;Matthias, T. ;VonLandenberg, P.; Oppermann,M. ;Helmke,K. and FÖrger, F.(2000).clinical relevance of antibodies against different phospholipids. Journal of Autoimmunity 15,A60.

Wramsby, M.L.., Sten-Linder, M.; and K Bremme, K. (2000). "Primary habitual abortions are associated with high frequency of Factor V Leiden mutation" American Society for Reproductive Medicine.5(6):455-458.

Wright, D.W.; Kellermann, A.L.; Hertzberg, V.S.; Clark, P.L.;Frankel, M..; Goldstein, F.C.; Salomone, J.P.;Dent, L.L.; Harris, O.A.; Ander, D.S.; Lowery, D.W.; Patel, M.M.; Denson, D.D.; Gordon, A.B.; Wald, M.M.; Gupta, S.; Hoffman, S.W. and Stein, D.G. (2007). "ProTECT: a randomized clinical trial of progesterone for acute traumatic brain injury". Ann. Emerg. Med.; 49 (4): 391–402.

Xiao, G.; Wei, J.; Yan, W.; Wang, W. and Lu, Z. (2008). "Improved outcomes from the administration of progesterone for patients with acute severe traumatic brain injury: a randomized controlled trial". Crit Care 12 (2): 61.

Zarutskiea, P.W.and Phillips, J.A. (2007). "Re-analysis of vaginal progesterone as luteal phase support (LPS) in assisted reproduction (ART) cycles". Fertility and Sterility 88 (1): 113.

Appendices

Appendix- I

Name:

Age:

Occupation:

Residence:

Rh-compatability:

G P A :

First abortion occur in 1st trimester◯ 2nd trimester◯ 3rd trimester◯

Second abortion occur in 1st trimester◯ 2nd trimester◯ 3rd trimester◯

Third abortion occur in 1st trimester◯ 2nd trimester◯ 3rd trimester◯

Forth abortion occur in 1st trimester◯ 2nd trimester◯ 3rd trimester◯

Fifth abortion occur in 1st trimester◯ 2nd trimester◯ 3rd trimester◯

Sixth abortion occur in 1st trimester◯ 2nd trimester◯ 3rd trimester◯

Seventh abortion occur in 1st trimester◯ 2nd trimester◯ 3rd trimester◯

History of infertility   –ve◯ +ve◯

　　　　　　　　Primary◯ secondary ◯

Mother side ◯ father side◯ both ◯

Is there any congenitale anomalies   yes◯ no◯

Past medical history:

◯hypertension

◯diabetic mellitus

◯deep venous thrombosis

◯asthma

Past surgical history

◯cervical circulage

◯fibroidactomy

Family history of abortion –ve◯ +ve◯

Mother◯

Sister◯

Ante◯

Appendices

Social history:

Smoking   Yes ◯ no ◯

Animals (cats) in home? Yes ◯ no ◯

Lab. Investigations:

1. Biochemical Investigations:

   1.1 Fasting blood sugar (FBS).

2 Heamatological Investigations:

   2.1 PCV.

   2.2 Hb concentrations.

3. Serological test

   3.1 Anti toxoplasma IgM antibodies

   3.2 Anti toxoplasma IgG antibodies

   3.3 Anti CMV IgM antibodies

   3.4 Anti CMV IgG antibodies

   3.5 Anti Rubella IgG antibodies

   3.6 Anti Rubella IgG antibodies

   3.7 Anticardiolipin IgM antibodies

   3.8 Anticardiolipin IgG antibodies

   3.9 Antiphospholipid IgM antibodies

   3.10 Antiphospholipid IgG antibodies

Appendix- I I

2.1 The Contents of the blood sugar kit

2.1.1 R1 . Monoreagent

Phosphate buffer 100 mmol/L pH 7.5, glucose oxidase > 10 KU/L, peroxidase > 2 KU/L, 4-aminoantipyrine 0.5 mmol/L, phenol 5 mmol/L.

2.1.2 (CAL) Glucose standard

Glucose 100 mg/dL (5.55 mmol/L).Organic matrix based primary standard. Concentration value is traceable to Standard Reference Material.

Appendices

2.2 Principle of fasting blood sugar (FBS) estimation

In the Tnnder reaction1, 2, the glucose is oxidized to D-gluconate by the glucose oxidase (GOD) with the formation of hydrogen peroxide. In the presence of peroxidase (POD), a mixture of phenol and 4-aminoantipyrine (4-AA) is oxidized by hydrogen peroxide, to form a red quinoneimine dye proportional to the concentration of glucose in the sample.

2.3 Procedure

Linear chemical instructions in Enzymatic colorimetric method for estimation of fasting blood sugar (Catalog Number:REF1129005) used(Young ,2000) were followed:

1. Bring reagents and sampls to room tempreture.
2. Pipettes into labeled tubes.

Tubes	Blank	Standard	CAL Standard
R1.mono Reagent	1.0 ml	1.0 ml	1.0 ml
Sample	—	10 µl	—
CAL Standard	—	—	10 µl

3. Mix and let the tubes stand 10 minutes at room temperatures or 5 minutes at 37 °c.
4. Read the absorbance (A) of the samples and the slandered at 500nmagainst the reagent blank.

2.4 Calculation

$$\frac{A\ Sample}{A}\ Standard\ Conc. = Glucose\ Conc.$$

Standard Conc. = 5.55 mmol/l

Appendix

3.1 Enzyme Linked Immunosorbent Assay (ELISA) procedure of anti-Toxoplasma (IgM,IgG) antibodies

Appendices

BioCheck instructions in Enzyme Linked Immunosorbent Assay (ELISA) of anti-toxoplasma IgG antibodies (Catalog Number: BC-1085), and IgM antibodies (Catalog Number: BC-1085) were used, (Voller *et al.*, 1976) were followed:

3.2 The contents of anti-toxoplasmosis (IgM &IgG) antibody kit

- Microliter Wells: Toxoplasma antigen-coated wells (12x8 wells)
- Enzyme Conjugate Reagent (red color): Red cap. 1 vial (12 ml)
- Sample Diluent (green color): 1 bottle (22 ml)
- Negative Calibrator: 0 IU/ml. Natural cap. (150 µl /vial)
- Cut-off Calibrator: 32 IU/ml. Yellow cap. (150 µl /vial)
- Positive Calibrator: 100 IU/ml. Red cap. (150 µl vial)
- Positive Calibrator: 300 IU/ml. Green cap. (150 vial)
- Negative Control: Range stated on label. Blue cap. (150 µl vial)
- Positive Control: Range stated on label. Purple cap. (150 µl vial)
- Wash Buffer Concentrate (20x):1 bottle (50 ml).
- TMB Reagent (One-Step): 1 vial (11 ml)
- Stop Solution: 1N HCl. Natural cap. 1 vial (11 ml)

3.3 The principle of the test

Purified Toxoplasma gondi antigen is coated on the surface of microwells. Diluted patient serum is added to the wells, & the Toxoplasma gondi IgG –specific antibodies ,if present, bind to the antigen. all unbound materials are washed away .HRP-conjugate is -added ,which bind to the antibody –antigen complex. Excess HRP-conjugate is washed off and a solution of TMB Reagent is added .the enzyme conjugate catalytic reaction is stopped at a specific time .the intensity of the color generated is proportional to the amount of (IgG or IgM)–specific antibody in the sample. The results are read by microwell reader compared in a parallel manner with calibrator and controls.

3.4 Specimen collection and preparation

1. Collect blood specimens and separate the serum.
2. Specemens may be refrigerated at 2-8 c° for up to 7 days or frozen for up to 6 months. Avoid repetitive freezing and thawing of serum sample.

Appendices

3.5 Reagent Preparation
1. All reagents should be allowed to reach room temperature (18-25 C°) before use.
2. Dilute 1 volume of wash Buffer (20x) with 19 volume of distilled water. Wash Buffer is stable for 1 month at 2-8 C°. Mix well before use.

3.6 Assay Procedure
1. Place the desired number of coated wells into the holder.
2. Prepare 1:40 dilution of test Samples, negative control, positive control, and calibrators by adding 5µl of the Sample to 200 µl of Sample Diluent. Mix well.
3. Dispense 100 µl of diluted sera, calibrators, and controls into the appropriate wells. For the reagent blank, dispense 100 µl Sample Diluent in 1A well position. Tap the holder to remove air bubbles from the liquid and mix well.
4. Incubate at 37 C° for 30 minutes.
5. At the end of incubation period, remove liquid from all wells. Rinse and flick the microtiter wells 5 times with diluted wash Buffer (1x).
6. Dispense 100 ml of Enzyme Conjugate to each well. Mix gently for 10 seconds.
7. Incubate at 37 C° for 30 minutes.
8. Remove Enzyme Conjugate from all wells. Rinse and flick the microtiter wells 5 times with diluted wash Buffer (1x).
9. Dispense 100 µl of TMB Reagent into each well. Mix gently for 10 seconds.
10. Incubate at 37 C° for 15 minutes.
11. Add 100 µl of Stop Solution (1N HCL) to stop reaction.
12. Mix gently for 30 seconds. It is important to make sure that all the blue color changes to yellow color completely.

Note: Make sure there are no air bubbles in each well before reading.

13. Read O.D. at 450 nm within 15 minutes with a microwell reader.

3.7 Calculation of the results
1. Calculate the mean of duplicate cut-off 932IU\ml) calibrator value xc.
2. Calculate the mean of duplicate positive control (xp), negative control (xn) and patient samples(xs).

Appendices

3. Calculate the toxoplasma (IgG ,IgM)index of each determination by dividing the mean values of each sample by calibrator mean value,xc.

3.8 Quantitative Estimation Of *Toxoplasma* (IgG ,IgM)

For a quantitative determination of anti –Toxoplasma (IgM,IgG) levels of positive specimens in IU\ml, OD of cut-off and positive calibrators are plotted on Y-axis in graph versus their corresponding anti-Toxoplasma (IgM,IgG) antibodies concentration of 0,32,100 and 300 IU\ml on X-axis. The Toxo (IgM, IgG) levels in patient sera are read off the graph using their individual OD values.

Appendix

4.1 Enzyme Linked Immunosorbent Assay (ELISA) procedure of anti- CMV (IgM,IgG) antibodies

BioCheck instructions in Enzyme Linked Immunosorbent Assay (ELISA) of anti-CMV IgG antibodies (Catalog Number: BC-1089), and IgM antibodies (Catalog Number: BC-1091) were used. The procedure that mentioned by Voller *et al.*, 1976 were followed.

4.2 The contents of anti-cytomegalovirus (IgM &IgG) antibody kit

-Microtiter strips: Strips with 8 breakable wells each coated with purified CMV antigen.

- Negative calibrator

-positive calibrator

-cut-off calibrator : CMV/IgG index= 1.0

-Negative control

-positive control

-Enzyme conjugate reagent: Anti-human-IgG-HRP (rabbit), 10 conjugated protein-containing buffer solution.

-Tetramethylbenzidin (TMB) substrate solution

-TMB stop solution: I N HCl.

-sample diluent: PBS buffer.

-Washing buffer concentrates (20x): PBS+Tween 20, 20x concentrate.
-Plastic foils: 2 pieces to cover the microtiter strips during the incubation

-Plastic bag: Resealable, for the dry storage of non-used strips.

Appendices

4.3 Preparation of samples and reagents

4.3.1 Samples

Before use, the patients' serum samples were diluted 1:40 with buffer serum diluents (the best chequre-board titration) (5µl of sample +200 µl buffer).

4.3.2 Wash Buffer

The wash buffer was diluted with distilled water 1 to 20 (10 ml concentrate + 190 ml distilled water).

4.4 Assay Procedure

1- A sufficient amount of microtiter wells was prepared for the standard controls and samples.

2- 1:40 dilutions of test samples, Negative Control, Positive Control, and Calibrator by adding 5µl of the sample to 200aµl of sample diluant were prepared.

3- 100µl of diluted sera, Calibrator, and Controls were dispensed into the appropriate wells of the strip.

4- The plates were covered with the enclosed foil and incubated at 37°c for 30 minutes.

5- At the end of incubation period, liquid was removed from all wells. the microtiter were rinsed and flicked 4 times with diluted wash bufferr (Ix) and then once with distilled water.

6- 100µl of enzyme conjugate was added to each well in sequence.

7- The plates were covered with enclosed foil and incubated for 30minutes at 37°C.

8- We rinsed and flicked the microtiter wells 4 times with diluted wash buffer (Ix) and then one time with distilled water.

9- 100µl of TMB reagent was added into each well.

10- The plates were covered with enclosed foil and incubated for 15minutes at 37 °c.

11- The reaction was stopped by adding 100 µl of TMB stop solution to each well.

12- The microtitter strips were shaken gently and the reading was taken at 450 nm within 15 minutes.

Appendices

4.5 Calculation of results

The results calculated according to (Cremer, 1985; Starr & Friedman, 1985;Voler & Bidwell, 1985).

1- Cutt-off calibrator value Xc was calculated.

2-Positive control (Xp), negative control (Xn) and patient samples (Xs) were calculated.

3- The CMV IgG and IgM Index of each determination by dividing the

Value of each sample (x) by calibrator value (Xc) were calculated.

4.6 Quantitative determination of CMV IgG & IgM antibodies

For a quantitative determination of anti-CMV IgG & IgM antibodies levels of posetive specimens in IU/ml, the O.D. of cut-off, negative, and posetive calibrators are plotted on the Y-axis of a graph against their corresponding anti-CMV IgG concentrations of 0, 1.2, 6, and 18IU/ml on the X-axis. The estimates of levels in patient sera are read off the graph using their individual O.D. values (Cremer, 1985; Starr &Friedman, 1985 ;Voler& Bidwell, 1985).

4.7 Interpretation of the results

The results of each sample were assessed according to (Cremer,1985 Starr & Friedman,1985;Voler& Bidwell,1985) as follows:

1-**Negative**: CMV IgG and IgM index less than 0.90 are seronegative for IgG and IgM antibody to CMV (<1.2 lU/ml).

2-**Equivocal**: CMV IgG and IgM Index between 0.91-0.99 are equivocal. sample should be retested.

3-**Posetive**: CMV IgG and IgM Index of 1.00 or greater, or IU value greater than seropositive (>1.2 lU/ml).

Appendix

5.1 Enzyme Linked Fluorescent Assay (ELFA) procedure of anti-Rubella (IgM,IgG) antibodies

BioMerieux instructions in Enzyme Linked Fluorescent Assay (ELFA) of antirubella IgM antibodies (Catalog Number: REF 30 214), and IgM antibodies (Catalog

Appendices

Number: REF 30 215) were used. The procedure that mentioned by Bellamy *et al.*(1986) ;Grangeot-Keros(1992) were followed.

5.2 The contents of anti-Rubella (IgM &IgG) antibody kit

30 RBM strips	STR	Ready-to-une
30 RBM SPRs 1 x30	SPR	Ready-to-use SPRs sensitized with anti- human u chain antibodies (goat) purified by affinity
RBM positive control1 x1 ml (liquid)	C 1	Ready-to-use Human* serum containing anti-Rubella IgM + 1 g/l sodium azide Index : the range is Indicated on the MLE card after the following mention "Control C1 (+) Test Value Range"
RBM negative control 1 x 1ml (liquid)	C 2	Ready-to-use. Human" serum negative for anti-Rubella IgM + 1 g/l sodium azide.
RBM Standard 1 x2ml (liquid)	S 1	Ready-to-usa Human* serum containing anti-Rubella IgM +1 g/l sodium azide.
1 MLE card		Specifications sheet containing the factory master calibration data required to calibrate the test
1 Package insert		

5.3 Principles

The assay principle combines the enzyme immunoassay method by capture with a final fluorescent detection (ELFA). The Solid Phase Receptacle (SPR) serves as the solid phase as well as the pipetting device for the assay. Reagents for the assay are ready-to-use and pre-dispensed in the sealed reagent strips.

All of the assay steps are performed automatically by the instrument. The reaction medium is cycled in and out of the SPR several times.

Appendices

After sample dilution, the IgM are captured by the polyclonal antibodies coating the interior of the SPR. Anti-rubella IgM are specifically detected by the inactivated rubella antigen, which is itself revealed by an alkaline phosphatase labeled anti-rubella monoclonal antibody (conjugate).

During the final detection step, the substrate (4-Methyl-ombelliferyl phosphate) is cycled in and out of the SPR. The conjugate enzyme catalyzes the hydrolysis of this substrate into a fluorescent product (4-Methyl-ombelliferone) the fluorescence of which is measured at 450 nm. At the end of the assay, an index is automatically calculated by the instrument in relation to the standard S1 stored in memory, and then printed out.

5.4 Test procedure

1. Only remove the required reagents from the refrigerator and allow them to come to room temperature for 30 minutes before use.
2. Use one RBM strip and one RBM SPR for each sample, control or standard to be tested. Make sure the storage pouch has been resealed after the required SPRs have been removed.
3. Type or select "RBM" on the instrument to enter the test code. The standard must be identified by "S1", and tested in duplicate. If the positive control is to be tested, it should be identified by "C1". If the negative control needs to be tested, it should be identified by C2.
4. Mix the standard, control and samples using a Vortex type mixer.
5. Pipette 100 µl of standard, sample or controls into the sample well.
6. Insert the SPRs and the Reagent Strips into the instrument. Check to make sure the color labeis with the assay code on the SPRs and the Reagent Strips match.
7. Initiate the assay as directed in the Operator's Manual. All the assay steps are performed automatically by the instrument. The assay will be completed within approximately 60 minutes
8. After the assay is completed, remove the SPRs and the strips from the instrument.
9. Dispose of the used SPRs and strips into an appropriate recipient.

Appendices

5.5 Results and interpretation

Once the assay is completed, results are analyzed automatically by the computer. Fluorescence is measured twice in the Reagent Strip s reading cuvette for each sample tested. The first reading is a background reading of the substrate cuvette before the SPR is introduced into the substrate The second reading is taken after the substrate has bee incubated with the enzyme remaining on the interior of the SPR. The RFV (Relative Fluorescence Value) is calculated by subtracting the background reading from the final result. This calculation appears on the result sheet The instrument calculates a test value (index) for each sample, which is the ratio between its RFV and that of the memorized standard.

This index and its interpretation appear on the result sheet.

Index i	Interpretation
i < 0.80	Negative
0.80 < i < 1.20	Equivocal
i > 1.20	Positive

Equivocal samples must be retested f the interpretation remains equivocal, a new sample must be collected 2 to 3 weeks later.

Interpretation of test results should be made taking into consideration the patient's history, and any other tests performed.

As no international standard is available for the determination of anti-Rubella IgM, the VIDAS RUB IgM reagent is calibrated against collection sera.

Appendix

6.1 Enzyme Linked Immunosorbent Assay (ELISA) procedure of antiphospholipid (IgM & IgG) antibody

Aeskulisa kit instructions in ELISA of antiphospholipid IgM (Catalog Number:REF-3224) and IgG (Catalog Number: REF-3225) antibody, The procedure that mentioned by Wöhrle *et al.*(2000) were followed.

6.2 The contents of antiphospholipid (IgM &IgG) antibody kit

-5x Sample Buffer   1 vial, 20 ml - 5x concentrated (capped white: yellow solution)

Appendices

Containing: Tris, NaCl, BSA, sodium azide < 0.1% (preservative)

-50x Wash Buffer   1 vial, 20 ml - 50x concentrated (capped white: green solution)

Containing: Tris, NaCl. Tween 20, sodium azide < 0.1% (preservative)

-Negative Control   1 vial, 1.5 ml (capped green: colorless solution)

Containing: Human serum (diluted), sodium azide < 0.1% (preservative)

-Positive Control   1 vial, 1.5 ml (capped red: yellow solution)

Containing: Human serum (diluted), sodium azide < 0 1% (preservative)

-Cut-off Calibrator   1 vial, 1.5 ml (capped blue: yellow solution)

Containing: Human serum (diluted), sodium azide < 0.1% (preservative)

- Calibrators   6 vials, 1.5 ml each 0, 3,10, 30,100, 300 GPL/ml or MPL/ml. (color increasing with concentration: yellow solutions)

Containing: Human serum (diluted), sodium azide < 0.1% (preservative)

-Conjugates   1 vial, 15 ml IgG (capped blue: blue solution)

1 vial,15 ml IgM (capped green: green solution)

Containing: Anti-human immunoglobulins conjugated to horseradish peroxidase

-TMB Substrate   1 vial, 15 ml (capped black)

Containing Stabilized TMB/H2O2

-Stop Solution 1 vial, 15 ml (capped white: colorless solution)

Containing: 1M Hydrochloric Add

-Microtiterplate   12x8 well strips with breakaway microwell

NoteThe contents of anticardiolipin (IgM &IgG) antibody kit is the same of the contents of antiphospholipid (IgM &IgG) antibody kit.

6.3 Principle of the test

Serum sample diluted 1:101 are incubated in the microplates coated with the specific antigen. Patient's antibodies, if present in the specimen, bind to the antigen. The unbound fraction is washed off in the following step. Afterwards anti-human immunoglobulin

Appendices

conjugated to horseradish peroxidase (conjugated) are incubated and react with the antigen-antibody complex of the samples in the microplates. Unbound conjugate is washed off in the following step. Addition of TMB-substrate generates an enzymatic colorimetric (blue) reaction, which is stopped by diluted acid (color changes to yellow). The rate of color formation from the chromogen is a function of the amount of conjugate bound to the antigen-antibody complex and this is proportional to the initial concentration of the respective antibodies in the patient sample.

6.3.1 Sample Collection, Handling and storage

Use preferentially freshly collected serum samples. Blood withdrawal must follow national requirements.

Do not use icteric, lipemic, hemolysed or bacterially contaminated samples. Sera with particles should be cleared by low speed centrifugation (<1000 x g). Blood samples should be collected in clean, dry and empty tubes. After separation, the serum samples should be used immediately, respectively stored tightly closed at 2-8 C° \35-46° F up to three days, or frozen at -20 C°\ -4° F for longer periods.

6.3.2 preparations prior to pipetting

Dilute the concentrated sample buffer 1:5 with distilled water. Dilute the concentrated wash buffer 1:50 with distilled water.

Samples:

Dilute serum samples 1:101 with sample buffer (1x).

Washing

Prepare 20 ml of diluted wash buffer (1x) per 8 wells or 200 ml for 96 wells

6.4 Assay procedure

1. Pipette 100µl of each patients diluted serum into the designated microwells.

2. Pipette 100 µl calibrators OR cut-off calibrator and negative and positive controls into the designated wells.

3. Incubate for 30 minutes at 20-32 c° \68-89.6° F.

4. Wash 3x with 300µl washing buffer (diluted 1:50).

5. Pipette 100µl conjugate into each well.

Appendices

6. Incubate for 30 minutes at 20 -32c° \68-89 °F.
7. Wash 3x with 300µl washing buffer (diluted 1:50).
8. Pipette 100µl TMB substrate into each well.
9. Incubate for 30 minutes at 20-32 c° \68-89.6° F, protected from intense light.
10. Pipette 100µl stop solution into each well, using the same order as pipetting the substrate.
11. Incubate 5 minutes minimum.
12. Agitate plate carefully for 5 second.
13. Read absorbance at 450 nm (optionally 450\620 nm) within 30 minutes.

6.5 Quantitative and Qualitative Interpretation

For the quantitative interpretation establish the standard curve by plotting the optical density (OD) of each calibrator (y-axis) with respect to the corresponding concentration values in U\ml (x axis).

For best results we recommend log \lin coordinates and 4 -parameter fit.

From the OD of each sample, read the corresponding antibody concentrations expressed in U\ml.

Normal range	Equivocal range	Positive results
<12 U\ml	12-18 U\ml	>18 U\ml

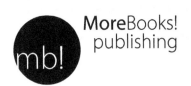
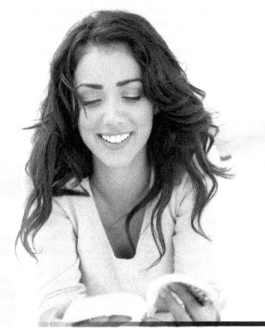

i want morebooks!

Buy your books fast and straightforward online - at one of world's fastest growing online book stores! Environmentally sound due to Print-on-Demand technologies.

Buy your books online at
www.get-morebooks.com

Kaufen Sie Ihre Bücher schnell und unkompliziert online – auf einer der am schnellsten wachsenden Buchhandelsplattformen weltweit! Dank Print-On-Demand umwelt- und ressourcenschonend produziert.

Bücher schneller online kaufen
www.morebooks.de

VDM Verlagsservicegesellschaft mbH
Heinrich-Böcking-Str. 6-8　　Telefon: +49 681 3720 174　　info@vdm-vsg.de
D - 66121 Saarbrücken　　　Telefax: +49 681 3720 1749　　www.vdm-vsg.de

Printed in the USA
CPSIA information can be obtained
at www.ICGtesting.com
LVHW042113120823
755063LV00007B/102